CLEAN & LEAN

FLAT TUMMY *FAST!*

THE HEALTHY WAY TO A TOTALLY TONED TUMMY IN 14 DAYS

James Duigan, fitness expert for The Times, and co-owner with Dalton Wong of Bodyism, London's premier fitness studio, is one of the world's top personal trainers. He is also the author of the bestselling Clean & Lean Diet. His many celebrity clients include Elle Macpherson, Rosie Huntington-Whiteley and Hugh Grant.

KYLE BOOKS

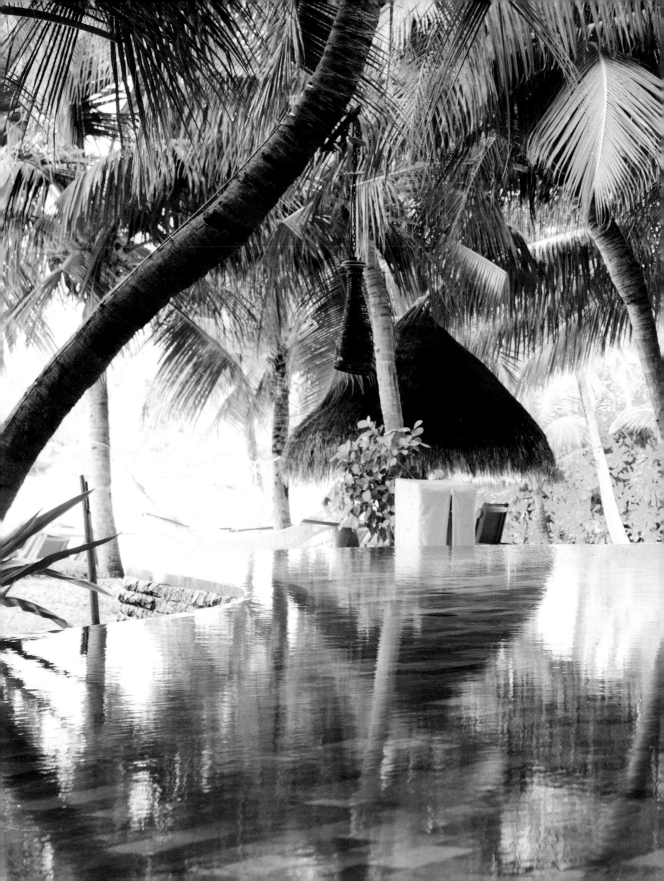

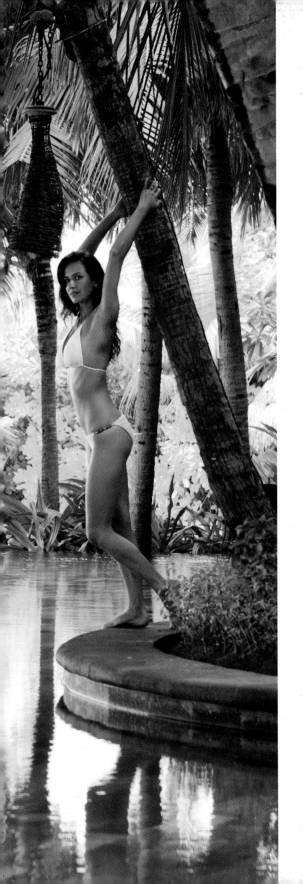

CLEAN & LEAN
FLAT TUMMY *FAST!*

THE HEALTHY WAY TO A
TOTALLY TONED TUMMY
IN 14 DAYS

JAMES DUIGAN
with Maria Lally

PHOTOGRAPHY BY
SEBASTIAN ROOS AND
CHARLIE RICHARDS
SHOT ON LOCATION AT
ONE&ONLY, REETHI RAH, MALDIVES

BODYISM: DALTON WONG AND
TIM PITTORINO

NUTRITION CONSULTANT:
ALICE SYKES PhD R.Nutr

KYLE BOOKS

This edition published in 2011 by
Kyle Books
23 Howland Street
London W1T 4AY
general.enquiries@kylebooks.com
www.kylebooks.com

ISBN 978 1 85626 987 2

First published in Great Britain in 2011 by
Kyle Cathie Ltd.

Editor Judith Hannam
Editorial Assistant Vicki Murrell
Design Dale Walker
Model Christiane Duigan
Location styling Emilie Lind
Recipe home economy Mary Jane Frost
Recipe styling Wei Tang
Copy editor Anne Newman
Proofreader Abi Waters
Production Gemma John

A Cataloguing in Publication record for this title is
available from the British Library.

Printed in China by C&C Offset Printing Co.

The information and advice contained in this book are
intended as a general guide. Neither the author nor the
publishers can be held responsible for claims arising from
the inappropriate use of any remedy or exercise regime.
Do not attempt self-diagnosis or self-treatment for serious
or long-term conditions before consulting a medical
professional or qualified practitioner. Do not begin any
exercise programme or undertake any self-treatment while
taking other prescribed drugs or receiving therapy without
first seeking professional guidance. Always seek medical
advice if any symptoms persist.

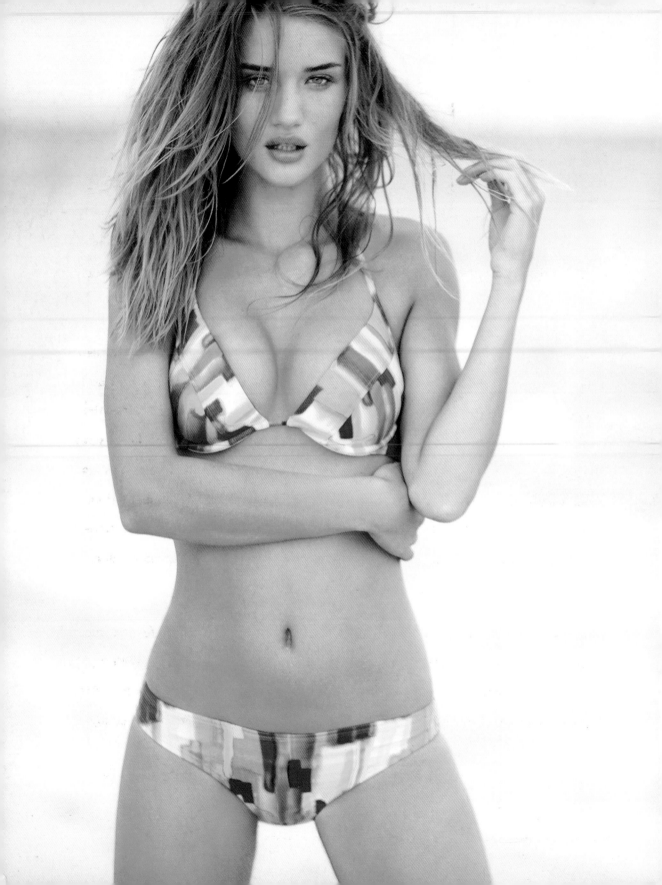

by Rosie Huntington-Whiteley

I was introduced to James two years ago, and I've trained with him ever since. He knows exactly how I want my body to look: lean, taut and strong, yet soft, curvy and feminine. Being healthy and feeling good, full of energy, glowing skin, these things are all really important to me. What I've learnt through working with James is that by focussing on creating a healthy body you can really achieve all of these things, faster than I ever thought possible. Oh, and by the way – nobody can get a stomach as flat as James can!

~

He keeps his workouts fresh and interesting so I never get bored, and he introduces new exercises all the time to keep my tummy – and body – in the best possible shape. I travel a lot for my job, so he's always coming up with ways for me to stay in shape and eat well when I'm staying in hotels or travelling between cities. Like most busy women, I can't go to the gym every single week and sometimes life just gets in the way of being able to maintain a routine every day and James understands this. So he gives me quick routines and funky shakes and supplements that keep my body looking good, even when I've got as little as 10 minutes a day to spend exercising. And when I need to get in shape fast – for a photoshoot or a film – he gets incredible results.

~

I love his Clean & Lean approach to diet and life – it's so simple and yet so effective. Once I had his 'Clean & Lean' mantra in my head, I found it easy to stay in shape with the right food, supplements and lifestyle choices, although I have to admit my favourite part is the yummy shakes he makes. So read on to find out just how easy it is to get the tummy – and the body – you've always dreamed of!

Rosie x

CHAPTER 1

THE CLEAN & LEAN WAY OF LIFE

THIS CHAPTER WILL HELP YOU TO DISCOVER:

1. WHAT 'CLEAN & LEAN' REALLY MEANS

2. HOW EASY IT IS TO BECOME CLEAN & LEAN

3. WHY SO MANY WOMEN HATE THEIR STOMACHS

4. HOW OUR COVER GIRL GOT HER FLAT TUMMY BY BECOMING CLEAN & LEAN

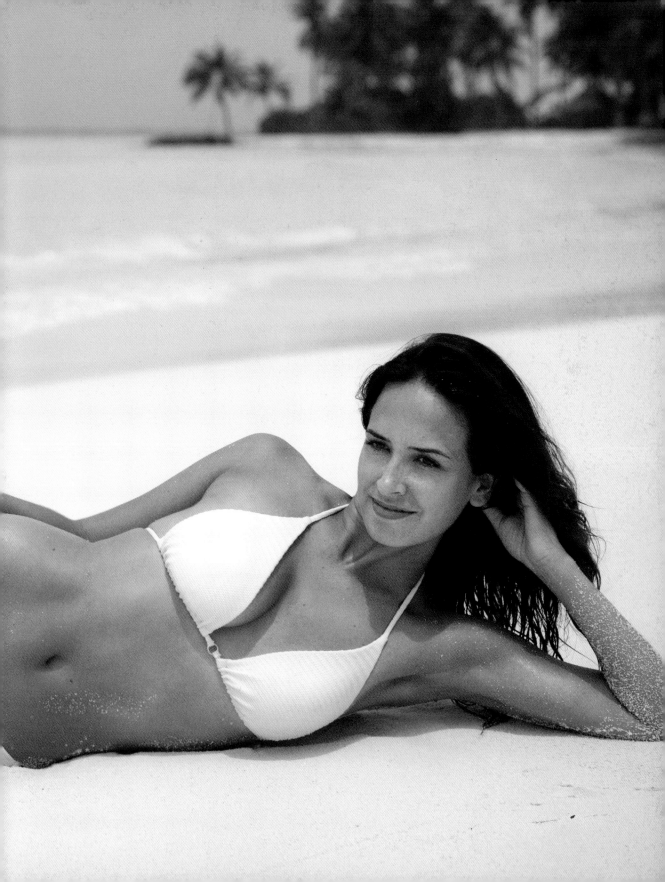

An amazing and wonderful transformation is possible for you right now. I have seen it happen thousands of times. This is the blueprint for a flat tummy fast. Don't let anything get in your way!

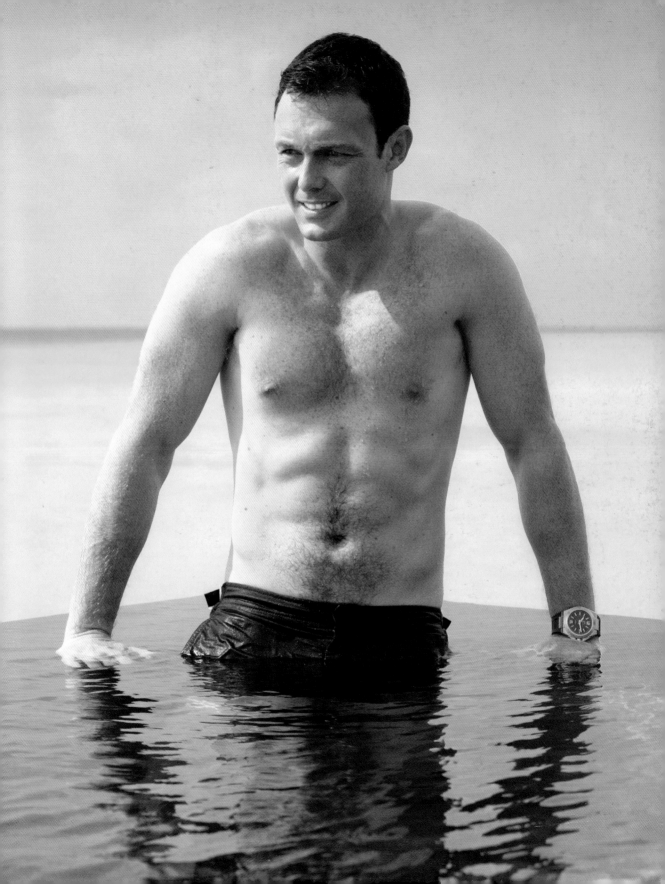

WHAT DOES CLEAN & LEAN REALLY MEAN?

As I explained in my first book, a body can never be lean unless it's clean. Toxins (I'll explain where they come from below) stop a body from becoming truly clean. That's because your body stores toxins in its fat cells. If you're dieting, but toxic, your body will slowly lose fat, but these toxins will have nowhere to go but back into your system. The result? You'll feel tired, you'll have headaches and you'll struggle with your energy levels. This is why most of us feel rotten within a few days of starting a diet. Your body decides it doesn't like feeling that way, so it holds on to fat in order to store the toxins. So if you're toxic, you'll always find it hard to lose weight. Ironically, many diets actually make us more toxic with all their low-fat/high-sugar foods. And so the cycle of yo-yo dieting continues. If you stick to 'Clean' foods – meaning toxin-free foods that are unprocessed and close to their natural state – then you'll lose weight easily and keep it off.

Clean foods

In a nutshell, clean foods:

* haven't changed much from their natural state – for example, an orange in a bowl looks like an orange hanging off a tree, whereas a crisp looks nothing like a potato – that's because it's been heavily processed and had all kinds of rubbish added to it
* don't need any added fake flavourings
* don't last for months and months – clean foods will go off in the fridge or cupboard pretty quickly as they don't contain preservatives
* don't contain more than 5 or 6 ingredients

✳ don't contain ingredients that you can't pronounce or that you don't recognise

✳ don't list sugar as either their main ingredient, or as one of their first 3 ingredients

✳ don't make you feel bloated, gassy or too full.

Where are toxins found?

These are the most common toxins:

✳ Sugar

✳ Alcohol

✳ Fizzy drinks

✳ Processed foods

✳ Processed 'diet' foods

✳ Excess caffeine

✳ Stress

My first book, the Clean & Lean Diet, became a bestseller, and I got thousands of letters from readers all over the world who loved the idea of slimming down all over, but the one thing they really, really wanted to know was how they could get a flat stomach fast – and how to keep it that way forever.

And, almost every client I've ever trained in my gym wants to know the same thing. Even the models. So in this book, I've taken the Clean & Lean approach and adapted it to target the tummy specifically. Following this plan will give you the stomach you've always dreamed of – one that is flat, feminine, toned and taut. There's no calorie counting, nor are there hundreds of sit-ups to do daily. In fact, in Chapter 6 I explain why sit-ups alone are not enough (see p. 91).

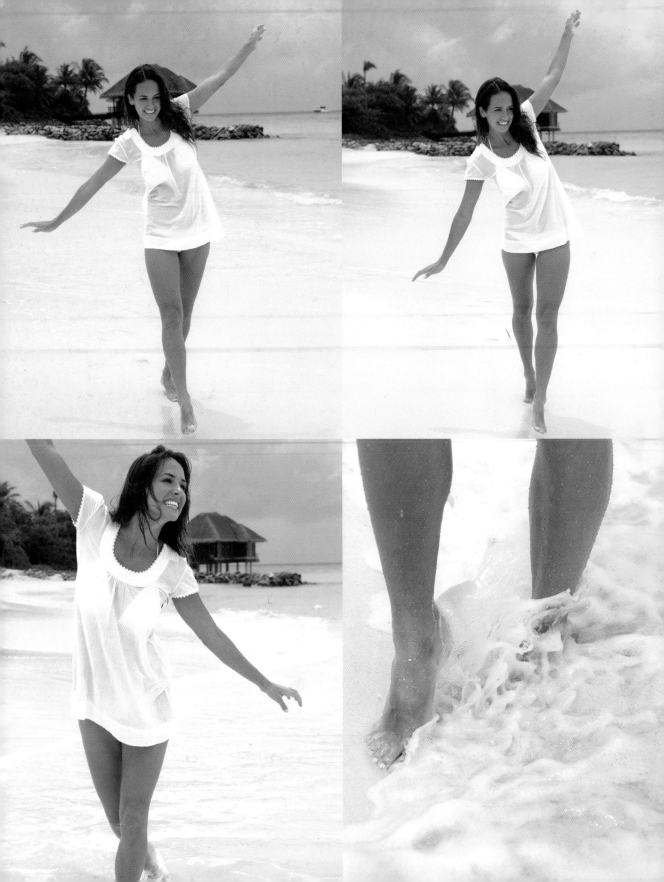

DISCOVER HOW EASY IT IS TO BECOME CLEAN & LEAN

All you need to do is follow the 14-day flat-tummy-forever eating plan detailed in Chapter 7 and, during that time, follow the easy exercise plan that starts on p. 69 (it only takes 10 minutes!). You can either read this book as you go along (being sure to finish it by the time the 14 days are up) or you can read the book first, and then start the 14-day plan straight after. Either way is fine. After the 14 days, I hope enough of the Clean & Lean approach will have sunk in for you to follow it thereafter as closely as your lifestyle allows. You don't have to stick to every single rule (although they're easy and you'll feel amazing if you do); just try to follow as many as you can and your stomach will look and feel amazing. In Chapter 9, there are some tips on keeping your tummy flat forever, and in Chapter 7 you'll also find delicious Clean & Lean tummy-flattening recipes for you to try.

Now, before we get going in earnest, here's a quick reminder of the Clean & Lean rules.

Sugar isn't so sweet

Sugar makes you fat. In fact, it converts to fat quicker than fat itself: sugary foods raise your insulin levels, which causes fat storage. Studies show that 40 per cent of the sugar you eat is converted straight to fat, and that's in a slim person. If you're already overweight, up to 60 per cent is converted straight to fat and stored around your stomach, waist and hips – meaning 60 per cent of that cupcake is heading straight to your tummy. Put simply – if you eat sugar every day, you'll always find it a struggle to lose weight and you'll never have a flat tummy.

Sugar also makes you more wrinkled. Your skin is supported by something called collagen – this is a protein found in the connective tissue of the skin. It's like a mattress that keeps the skin plump, bouncy and firm to the touch and young looking. Over time, however, collagen breaks down causing a sagging, wrinkled appearance, and sugar ultimately speeds up the breakdown. So that cupcake won't just add inches to your waistline – it will add wrinkles and years to your face too.

Sugar also leaches vitamins from your body, and a body starved of vitamins becomes hungry. That's why overweight people are always hungry – they don't eat enough vitamin-rich food and are actually malnourished. Toxic foods like sugar will never satisfy you or fill you up. Plus, sugar also makes you tired, lowers libido and weakens the immune system.

So why do we love it so much? Sugar is physically and emotionally addictive. It's physically addictive because it has the same effect on the brain as pain-killing medication, such as morphine, producing an almost instant feeling of pleasure and satisfaction, and giving you an energy hit. But this energy is all too fleeting – sugar raises your blood-sugar levels too quickly, causing them to crash, and leaving you exhausted.

It's emotionally addictive too. Most sugar fans grew up viewing it as a treat or a reward – say, in the form of birthday cakes or a bag of sweets for getting good grades at school. And now, as adults, they still see it that way – 'rewarding' themselves with ice cream after a bad break-up or a cupcake with a friend over coffee after a tough week at work. Sugar has always been associated with making us feel better. But look beyond the pretty pink icing on the cupcake and you'll see sugar for what it is – a fattening toxin that makes you wrinkled, tired and malnourished, while adding a layer of flesh on to your tummy.

*remember
Sugar is like a nuclear fat bomb exploding all over your body.

Cut the CRAP*

* Caffeine, refined sugar, alcohol and processed foods

The 4 main toxins that cause our bodies to cling to fat:
✳ caffeine ✳ refined sugar ✳ alcohol ✳ processed foods.

CAFFEINE

Caffeine is OK in small doses. A cup of coffee a day won't do you much harm, and some studies suggest it can even help with fat burning. The same goes for tea. Green tea – which also contains caffeine – is an even better fat burner. I let my clients drink up to 6 cups of green tea a day (not in the evening though, as it can stop you sleeping). The trouble with caffeine is, too much of it causes stress to your body. And, as you'll learn in Chapter 3, too much stress dumps a ring of fat around your middle.

REFINED SUGAR

I've already covered refined sugar on page 15, and I'll talk more about why it makes your tummy fat in Chapter 2 (see pp. 20–27).

ALCOHOL

Alcohol is full of sugar, and as a result, makes you fat around the middle. It stimulates the production of the hormone oestrogen in your bloodstream, which promotes fat storage (specifically around your waist and tummy). In addition to this, the liver is a fat-burning organ, but when it's busy processing alcohol, it stops burning fat. Alcohol also decreases muscle growth, leaving you podgy and out of shape. I see so many women with what I call a 'wine waist' – a thick waist and a swollen, squidgy tummy as a result of regularly drinking wine 3 or 4 days or evenings a week.

PROCESSED FOODS

I'm going to talk more about processed foods in Chapter 2; in a nutshell though, they go against every Clean & Lean rule there is. The less a food has been altered, the 'cleaner' it is and the better it is, therefore, for our health and waistlines. Clean foods are very close – if not the same – as their natural state, whereas processed foods are far from it. They are usually made in factories, stripped of their natural goodness and pumped full of man-made preservatives and additives to make them look appetising and – crucially – last longer.

FOODS TO AVOID

✳ Tinned foods
✳ White bread, pasta and rice
✳ Processed meats
✳ Breakfast cereals
✳ Frozen ready meals
✳ Frozen chips, wedges, etc.
✳ Packets of dried pasta
✳ Packaged cakes, biscuits, muffins
✳ Chocolate, sweets and crisps

Fat phobia makes you fat

New clients always tell me, 'I have hardly any fat in my diet'. Yet this is usually one of the reasons why they need to see me in the first place.

Don't be afraid of fat – I can't stress this enough. Of course, when I say this, I'm talking about good fat – found in nuts, avocados, oily fish and oils. I'm not talking about bad fat, also known as trans fats.

Good fats should be eaten every single day. They encourage your body to burn fat around your middle,

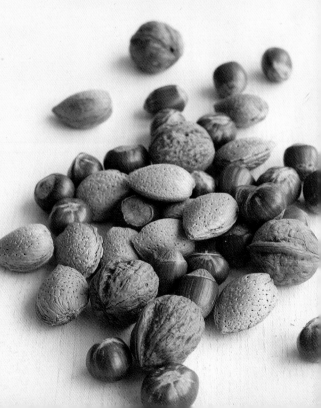

giving you a nice, flat tummy. They help your body to absorb vitamins and minerals more efficiently. So whenever you have a salad, always add some good fat to it – whether you drizzle it with olive oil or sprinkle over some chopped nuts or seeds. That way, your body will better absorb all those lovely nutrients from the vegetables.

Eating good fats every day will also banish the following all-too-common symptoms:

* Inability to concentrate
* Sluggishness
* Feeling physically full but still hungry
* Craving something sweet after a meal
* A mid-afternoon energy dip
* Difficulty waking up in the morning
* A feeling of lethargy and fatigue

The cheat meal

This is my clients' favourite Clean & Lean rule! Once a week, I let them have a 'cheat meal'. This can be anything from a plate of creamy pasta to a huge slice of chocolate cake with cream. It can only be one meal (i.e. breakfast, lunch or dinner and one course of a meal – not a starter, main and dessert) and it can only be once a week. This doesn't just help to keep you on track with your diet, it also actually speeds up your metabolism. When you're eating clean foods all the time and generally being good, your metabolism stays nice and steady. However, every once in a while you need to give it a good boost. And eating more than usual does just that: your metabolism goes into shock and starts working overtime to burn off the extra food. This doesn't work if you eat rubbish all the time, but a once-a-week cheat meal will improve fat burning, plus it will mean you can still eat your favourite foods (in moderation).

The bath that helps you lose weight

Like the cheat meal, another easy Clean & Lean rule is the Epsom salts bath. Lots of my model clients take one just before a bikini shoot. Basically, you add one or two mugs of Epsom salts (you can buy these in most pharmacies) to a hot bath – not too hot, as you want to be able to sit in it comfortably. Epsom salts are an ancient remedy for drawing out toxins. Taking 1 or 2 of these baths a week will speed up your weight loss.

WHY SO MANY WOMEN HATE THEIR TUMMIES

Nearly every woman who has ever stepped foot inside my gym, has told me they hate their tummy, and countless studies say it's the least-favoured body part.

There are a number of reasons why women in particular store fat around their tummies. Men tend to crave high-protein foods, such as steak and eggs, which feed muscles rather than fat cells, while women have sugar and fat cravings (chocolate, cake, etc) that often intensify at specific times in the menstrual cycle and result in a short-lived happier mood. However, this doesn't last and the excess of sugar tends to deposit fat all over their stomach and love-handle areas.

Secondly, there is a condition called visceroptosis, which is more common in women than in men. It involves a sinking of the abdominal organs, which results in a tummy paunch. It's basically what happens when the body's natural girdle (the muscles that make the tummy flat) become defective. The condition can be caused by a loss of abdominal muscle tone, constipation and eating foods that inflame the gut and intoxicate the intestines (predominantly processed foods). Most cases can be cured with cleaning up your diet, improving your posture and maintaining good abdominal strength from the right exercises.

The third reason females may have a distended tummy is if they become pregnant again before their body has fully restored its optimal muscle strength, proper posture and ideal body weight. With multiple pregnancies, the body can forget what it should feel like. Waiting two years between pregnancies can prevent this paunch, as can good core conditioning in between pregnancies. I train lots of new mums, and a post-pregnancy tummy-flattening plan involving proper nutrition and exercise can see the return of a pre-baby body in no time at all (see pp. 44 and 53).

So, whether you're a new mum who wants her old tummy back, you've struggled with your stomach all your life, or it's simply not as flat as it used to be, read on and discover how to achieve a Clean & Lean flat tummy – fast!

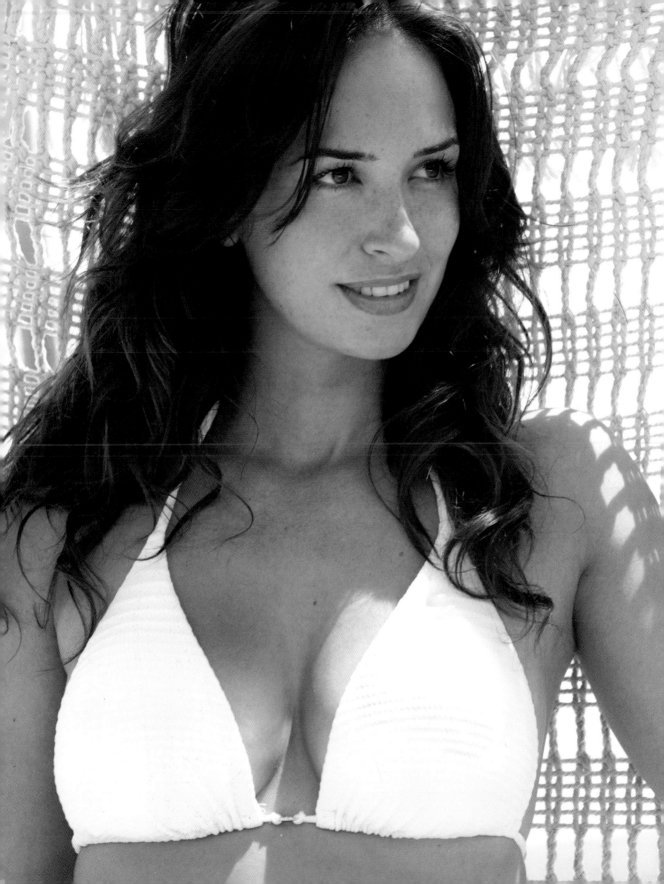

HOW OUR COVER GIRL GOT HER FLAT TUMMY BY BECOMING CLEAN & LEAN

The cover star of this book – and the original Clean & Lean book – is my wife, Christiane. Believe it or not, there was a time when she didn't like her tummy. Then she met me – I told her all about my Clean & Lean diet, she became a total convert and the results speak for themselves! Here's her story:

As a teenager I was naturally skinny and didn't have to watch what I ate. Growing up in Australia, they called me the 'Queen of Lollies' because I loved lollies and sweets so much. Then, when I hit 23, things started to change. The weight crept on, especially around my tummy and waist, and I couldn't get away with all those sweets and lollies any more.

I arrived in the UK a year later, and was nearly 9 kilograms heavier than I had been. I started to follow every fad diet that was out there. They were usually very restrictive and full of low-fat diet products. I went to the gym most days and did lots of cardio, but the weight was still stubbornly clinging on. Like most women, I hated my tummy the most. It was podgy and wobbly and no amount of sit-ups seemed to tone it up.

I was always stressing about my weight, which I now know is one of the worst diet downfalls. As I learned from James, stressing about fat can actually make you fatter. I was stuck in a cycle of diets: I'd lose a bit, then put it back on the minute I relaxed my diet or exercise. I was looking for a diet that didn't feel like a diet – I wanted to eat healthily, exercise a bit, but still live normally and not feel like I was constantly depriving myself.

Then I met James, but I didn't know he was a personal trainer at first. I told him, just in passing, that I wanted to shape up, so he suggested I try his Clean & Lean programme. He told me all about clean foods, the amazing Bodyism supplements to help my body stay clean and lean and suggested I cut back on the cardio and incorporate some stress-busting stretch circuits and massages into my workouts, plus some weights. Beforehand I'd been terrified of weights, and just did cardio gym classes and ran and ran on the treadmill. I thought weights would bulk me up, but James showed me how they actually burn serious amounts of fat in a very short space of time, and really tone and tighten a woman's body. And the rest is history. Despite exercising less and eating more, the extra weight just fell off in a few months.

The best part of all is that my tummy became very, very flat. All those diet foods I'd been eating, and the stress I'd been feeling, were the reasons behind my podgy tummy. But once I was eating and living Clean & Lean, my stomach really sucked itself in and my waist got narrower. My weight didn't fluctuate; it just stayed the same. Before the photo shoot for the book and before my wedding, I went on the 6-Day Tummy Transformer and even though it's tough it gets my tummy trim and unbloated quickly in time for a special occasion. And my energy levels have soared. I rarely feel tired during the day now because I'm not on a constant high or low from sugar. My concentration and memory are better too.

All that happened 3 years ago, but I still follow the Clean & Lean approach today. And the best bit? I get to eat my cheat meal of hot chocolate pudding every week and still look like this!

Christiane Duigan

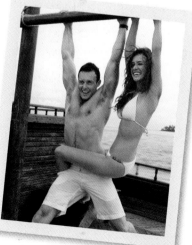

CHAPTER 2

EAT YOUR WAY TO A FLATTER TUMMY

THIS CHAPTER WILL HELP YOU:

DISCOVER THE FOODS THAT WILL KEEP YOUR TUMMY FLAT

... AND THE ONES THAT WILL KEEP IT FAT

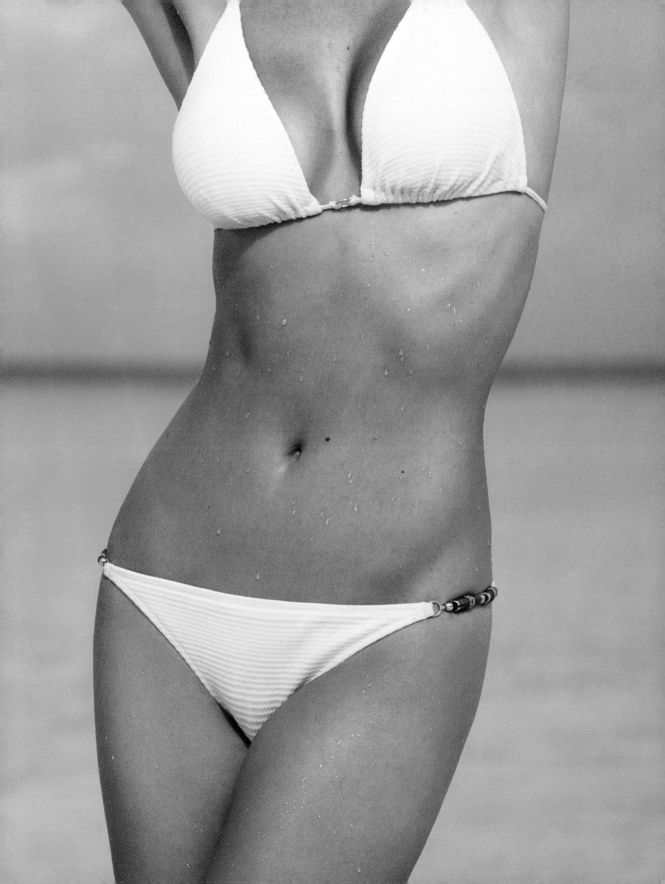

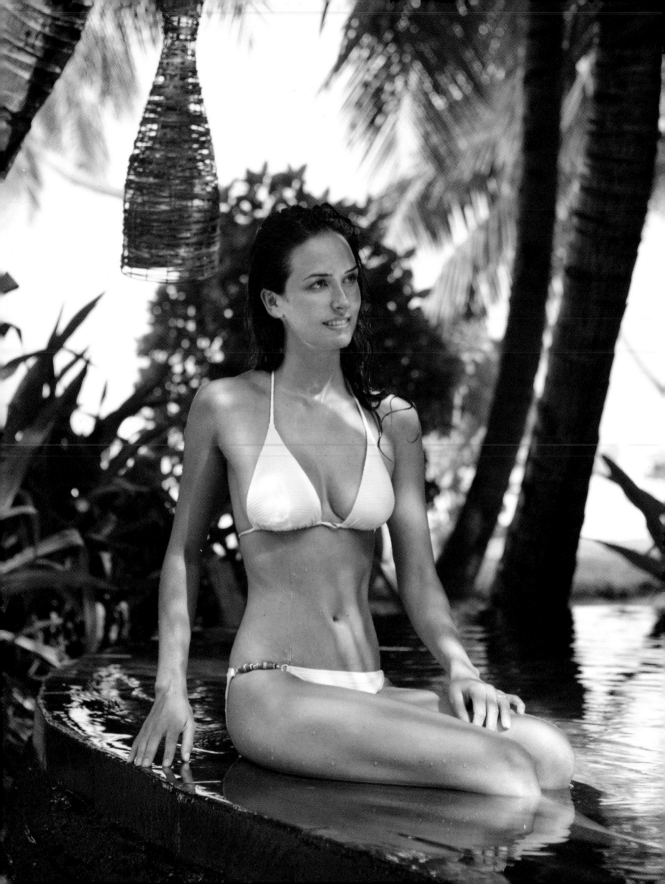

In the following chapters, I'll be talking about what contributes to making your tummy fat (including stress and too little sleep) and what makes it nice and flat (good sleeping habits and a weekly back massage – yes really!). But the biggest contributor of all is, unsurprisingly, what you eat. But it's not just a case of being overweight, therefore you have a fat stomach. Even a slim person can have a protruding, swollen and fat stomach if they eat the wrong food. In this chapter I'm going to tell you the changes you need to make to your diet in order to get a flat stomach... fast!

Become less acidic

Now this gets a bit science-y, but if you want a flat stomach then you need to become less acidic and more alkaline. The best way to become alkaline (or to achieve 'an alkaline state') is to eat plenty of alkaline foods and – where possible – reduce acidic ones.

Acidic food stresses out your body, and stops you creating lots of lovely lean muscle, which makes you look amazingly toned and speeds up your metabolism. Too much acidic food also inflames your body, especially your gut, which is why people with acidic diets tend to have a distended, bloated little 'pooch' tummy. This is important, so listen up: Once your tummy is flat and you have balanced yourself out, you can ease up on being so strict with what you eat. In the meantime, stick with it, your body will thank you.

Here are some signs that your body may be too acidic, particularly if you suffer from two or more symptoms:
* You have an inflamed, sticky-out stomach
* You frequently have problems with your digestive system – such as indigestion, IBS (Irritable Bowel Syndrome), bloating etc.
* You frequently get colds
* You have low energy levels
* You suffer from headaches
* Your joints often ache
* You're prone to nasal congestion

However, I'm not saying you have to eat an entirely alkaline diet. In moderation, some acidic foods are great and necessary. The key is to tip the balance in favour of alkaline foods and away from the acidic ones. As a general rule, make 70 per cent of the foods in your diet alkaline, and 30 per cent acidic. For example, for each serving of protein on your plate have 2 big portions of veggies.

ALKALINE

Try to include as many in your diet as possible:
* Chicken – most meats are acidic, but chicken is actually alkalising.
* Nuts
* Berries
* Avocadoes
* Lemons (this might confuse you – after all lemons are acidic, surely? Well, no – they may taste acidic but they're actually very alkalising and calm the body)
* Limes (ditto)
* Grapefruits (ditto)
* Tomatoes
* Watermelons
* Artichokes
* Asparagus
* Beetroot
* Broccoli
* Brussels sprouts
* Cabbage
* Carrots
* Cauliflower
* Celery
* Courgettes
* Cucumber
* Green beans
* Kale
* Leeks
* Lettuce
* Onions
* Peas
* Radishes
* Spinach
* Swedes
* Watercress

ACID

* All fruits aside from those listed left. I'm not saying don't eat fruit – far from it. It can make up 30 per cent of a meal (for example, berries with yogurt and nuts).
* Turkey
* Beef
* Lamb
* Pork
* Seafood (excluding oily fish, such as salmon)
* Cheese
* Cream
* Eggs
* Ice-cream
* Milk
* Yogurt
* White pasta
* White/wholemeal bread
* Sweets/candy
* Chocolate
* Biscuits
* Artificial sweeteners
* Refined sugar
* All fizzy drinks
* Coffee
* Tea
* Alcohol
* Fruit juice
* Condiments
* Honey
* Margarine
* Corn oil
* Vegetable oil
* Sunflower oil
* Trans fat*
* Peanuts
* Cashew nuts
* Pistachio nuts

Your body can also become acidic if you're too stressed – in chapter 3, I'll explain how you can become less stressed.

AVOID PESTICIDES!

Pesticides are basically poisons that are sprayed onto foods to kill off insects. The farmers use low enough levels so as not to kill humans. However, they're still a toxin and best avoided. The following are a list of fruits and vegetables (all healthy, clean and lean) that are typically sprayed with pesticides. I've listed them in order of their 'pesticide load' – so the ones at the top of the list contain more pesticides than those at the bottom. Don't avoid the foods at the top of the list – but it's important to remember that they typically contain more pesticides so ideally buy them organically. Or give them a good rinse before you eat them. This isn't so important with foods that have thick, tough skins that aren't eaten (such as bananas). But it's very important to wash foods with thin skins that you do eat (such as grapes and berries). Just think about it – if you sprayed something (let's say hairspray for example) onto a banana, once you'd peeled and eaten it, you'd barely taste the hairspray. But if you sprayed a strawberry with hairspray you'd taste it because the skin is so thin (and edible). Remember – less pesticides = a cleaner, therefore leaner body.

* Peaches
* Apples
* Peppers
* Celery
* Nectarines
* Strawberries
* Cherries
* Kale
* Lettuce
* Grapes
* Carrots
* Pears
* Collard Greens
* Spinach
* Potatoes
* Green Beans
* Squash
* Cucumbers
* Raspberries

* Plums
* Oranges
* Cauliflower
* Tangerines
* Mushrooms
* Bananas
* Cantaloupe melons
* Cranberries
* Honeydew melons
* Grapefruits
* Sweet potatoes
* Tomatoes
* Broccoli
* Watermelons
* Papaya

For a comprehensive list of these foods, please log on to bodyism.com.

A WORD OF WARNING ABOUT TRANS FATS

Trans fat is a re-heated oil that's pumped into food to prolong its shelf life and add flavour. Yuck! It's a money making thing – after all, food that's pumped full of trans fats lasts for ages so the food manufacturers make less of a loss on their products. Trans fats have been linked to obesity, some cancers and even infertility and are found in:

* Biscuits
* Muffins
* Some margarines

* Pastries
* Crisps
* Mousses

Always check the label for 'trans fats'. It also goes under the following names: 'Hydrogenated oil', 'Hydrogenated Vegetable Fat' or 'Partially Hydrogenated Vegetable Oil'.

THE 7 QUESTIONS I ASK ALL MY CLIENTS

The majority of my female clients come to me extremely frustrated, complaining, 'James, I eat really well and exercise hard but I still can't get rid of this paunch belly.' After I clean up their diet (by cutting the CRAP; see chapter 1) and make sure they know how to exercise and work their abdominals properly (see chapter 6), I sometimes find there's still a stubborn paunch tummy protruding, usually just below their belly button. When this happens, I ask them whether:

They currently take, or have ever taken

1. Antibiotics – if so, how many times and when was the last time?
2. The oral contraceptive pill – if so, for how long and did they notice any side-effects when they started taking it?
3. Steroids for medical or any other reason?

They have been exposed to

4. Radiation (X-rays and radiation therapies)

They consume

5. Chlorinated water? (This includes all forms of tap water.)
6. Refined sugars and other refined foods? If so, how often, how much and exactly what types of foods or products over the past two years?

They have suffered from

7. Poor digestion, constipation, or experienced stress that affects the digestion?

As healthy and hard working as my clients are, they are often answer yes to several of these questions. I then explain how all of these things severely disrupt the microflora colony in their digestive tract. You see, the ideal ratio of friendly bacteria in a healthy human gut is 85 per cent friendly bacteria and 15 per cent harmful bacteria. However many studies show that too many people in the West have this ratio the other way around – 85 per cent unfriendly bacteria and just 15 per cent friendly bacteria. Common signs that your gut flora is unbalanced, (which chances are it is) include:

● Bloating
● Indigestion
● Frequent and/or smelly flatulence
● Abdominal distension or discomfort
● Diarrhoea and/or constipation
● Food intolerances and allergies

In short, if your stomach doesn't feel fantastic or if it looks or feels noticeably different (swollen, sore, bloated, etc) after eating certain foods then it may be time you cleaned up your gut in order to get your stomach really flat by repopulating your gut with billions of friendly bacteria. To do this you must first eliminate all the foods, chemicals and products that cause the bad bacteria to breed. These include:

✻ Tap water. Buy a filter jug instead and drink from that.
✻ Non organic meat. Farm animals are fed antibiotics to keep diseases down so when you eat meat, you take in these antibiotics. Make sure all of your meat is organic. If money is an issue, eat meat less often and buy better quality for the times when you do eat it.
✻ Alcoholic drinks. These kill friendly probiotics, encouraging harmful bacteria and yeast overgrowth (they're also packed with sugar, which makes you fat).
✻ Antibiotics. These directly kill all bacteria (friendly and unfriendly) in your intestinal tract, which is why probiotics are recommended after taking antibiotics.
✻ Birth control pills and many other everyday over-the-counter-drugs cause damage to intestinal flora and to the tissue in the intestinal wall, which can weaken it. They can also inflame the abdominal wall. Both of these things can lead to a paunch. So keep all unnecessary medications to an absolute minimum.

Once your digestive system is weakened, the bad bacteria can breed faster and it can take years to undo. However, don't start stressing just yet because I have flattened even the most stubborn of stomachs when I put their owners on my Clean & Lean Flat Tummy plan.

In a nutshell, you need to stop feeding the bad bacteria and start feeding the good, friendly bacteria with both pre- and probiotics. You also need to stop eating refined sugar, processed foods, taking unnecessary over-the-counter-medications*, drinking tap water and alcohol, and ideally find alternative methods of birth control other than the contraceptive pill**.

*When I say 'unnecessary', I mean headache pills for gentle headaches that could be dealt with by sleeping more, drinking more water or reducing stress. I don't mean life-saving or health-boosting medication. Always speak to your doctor before coming off medication.
**Always speak to your doctor or family planning nurse before changing your contraception.

*top tip
Probiotics and prebiotics are an amazing way of improving your gut health immediately.

WHERE IS REFINED SUGAR FOUND?

* White sugar (the type you might put in your tea)
* Fruit juices
* White, non-organic pasta, bread and rice
* Alcohol
* Cakes, sweets, biscuits, ice cream
* Foods marketed as 'low fat', including cereal bars, muffins, cereals and energy drinks.
* Any ingredient ending in 'ose' (such as sucrose, glucose, maltose, lactose, dextrose and fructose).
* Anything with the following in the ingredients list:

* Syrup	* Maltose
* High fructose corn syrup	* Xylitol
* Brown sugar	* Sorbitol
* Cane syrup	* Mannitol
* Sucrose	* Erythritol
* Glucose	* Aspartame
* Dextrose	* Saccharin
* Fructose	* Nutrisweet
* Sucanat	* Splenda
* Turbinado sugar	* Cyclamate
* Beet sugar	* Sucralose
* High fructose corn syrup	* Acesulfame-Kneotame.

Instead, you need to start eating lots of foods containing pro- and prebiotics, as this will encourage the growth of friendly bacteria in your gut.

Probiotics are found in:
* Sauerkraut (fermented cabbage)
* Kimchi (Korean spicy cabbage)
* Miso
* Fermented dairy products such as acidophilius milk (available at all good health stores but make sure its not the high sugar 'pretend' health drinks)
* Yogurt
* Some soft cheeses
* cultured buttermilk
* Soured cream
* Yogurt products (look for 'live cultures added' in the ingredients list or on the front of the packet)

Prebiotics are found in:
* Bananas
* Berries
* Asparagus
* Garlic
* Tomatoes
* Onions
* Spinach
* Kale
* Lentils
* Kidney beans
* Chickpeas
* Black beans
* Oats
* Unrefined wheat
* Unrefined barley

Vitamin C makes pre- and probiotics more effective, so tuck into vitamin C-rich foods every day. These include:
* Kiwi fruit
* Oranges
* Sweet potatoes
* Broccoli
* Brussels sprouts
* Peppers
* Strawberries
* Papaya
* Grapefruit
* Tomatoes

WHAT ARE PRE- AND PROBIOTICS?

Probiotics and prebiotics are not the same things. Probiotics are live microorganisms, known as friendly bacteria, and are responsible for several important biological functions, including boosting your digestion, reducing levels of 'bad' gut bacteria and strengthening the immune system. Prebiotics are non-digestible ingredients found in certain foods that stimulate the growth of friendly bacteria in the gut. They both work together to boost gut health, so you need both, either through supplementation or food.

*top tip
For a full list of these foods, please log on to bodyism.com.

SUPPLEMENTS AND PROBIOTICS:

There are several supplements out there. However, I find the best ones are those that contain at least 3 billion to 5 billion live organisms (check the label). Another factor when buying a probiotic is it should contain several different strands of bacteria, including Lactobacillus bulgaricus, Lactobacillus acidophilus, Streptococcus thermophilus and bifidobacteria. Kefirs, such as coconut kefir or goat's milk kefir are a fantastic natural probiotic. Quick tip: your probiotic supplements should always be refrigerated. Prebiotic supplements should be take around 15 minutes BEFORE a meal and probiotic supplements should be taken AFTER a meal. Bodyism has a great pre- and probiotic, otherwise ask in your local health store for a recommendation.

WHY PROBIOTICS HELP YOU LOSE BELLY FAT

An important part in losing weight around your stomach is to ensure that your digestive system is working to its best ability, and this is exactly what probiotics do. They also help your body absorb health-boosting nutrients from your food better. So remember – unless your gut is as healthy as it can be, then your stomach will always be fat. Your body will become overloaded with toxins and you'll always find losing weight a struggle.

Health benefits of pre- and probiotics include:

1. Reduced cancer risk
2. Lower 'bad' cholesterol levels
3. Increased vitamin absorption from your foods
4. Boosted immune system
5. Steady blood sugar levels
6. Less constipation and diarrhoea
7. Reduced risk of bowel disorders

OTHER WAYS TO EAT YOUR WAY TO A FLATTER STOMACH

● Don't overcook your food as you'll kill off or reduce the number of nutrients it contains. Try to make sure around 50 per cent of the food on your plate is raw. If you can stomach it eat all your vegetables raw. If not, see chapter 7 for ways on cooking your vegetables while still retaining as many of their nutrients as possible.

● Don't buy cheap meat – organic meat is more expensive, but it also contains less toxic junk like antibiotics (given to non-organic animals). I tell my clients to buy everything organic, but if you can only afford one organic thing make sure it's meat.

● Don't eat foods that weaken your abdominal wall, as this will make it slack and lead to a protruding stomach. Foods that can weaken your abdominal wall often contain gluten. Lots of people are gluten intolerant and it inflames their bowel which makes it look bigger, especially just below the belly button. Foods containing gluten include:

* Bread and pasta (unless otherwise stated)
* Most breakfast cereals
* Muffins
* Pastries
* Baked goods
* Pizza bases
* Pie crusts
* Biscuits
* Cakes
* Croissants
* Bagels
* Alcohol made from grains – ie, beer, whisky, bourbon and liqueurs
* Cheese spread
* Ketchup
* Processed meats
* Margarine
* Oats
* Salad dressings
* Sausages
* Seasoning mixes
* Semolina
* Soups – apart from home made ones
* Soy sauce and most Chinese sauces
* Sweets which contain grain (stabilisers made from gluten)

● Avoid sugar, in all its forms, as it leads to an increase of fat around your middle section (waist and stomach).

● Make sure you eat enough fibre. A lack of fibre will lead to inflammation in the bowel. Eat plenty of vegetables (ideally raw ones) and drink at least 2 litres of still, room temperature water every day.

CHAPTER 3

WHY STRESS MAKES YOUR TUMMY FAT

THIS CHAPTER WILL TEACH YOU:

1. HOW TO EAT YOURSELF LESS STRESSED
2. HOW TO EXERCISE YOURSELF LESS STRESSED
3. HOW TO HAVE A STRESS DETOX
4. ALL YOU NEED TO KNOW ABOUT
STRESS-BUSTING MINERALS AND HERBS

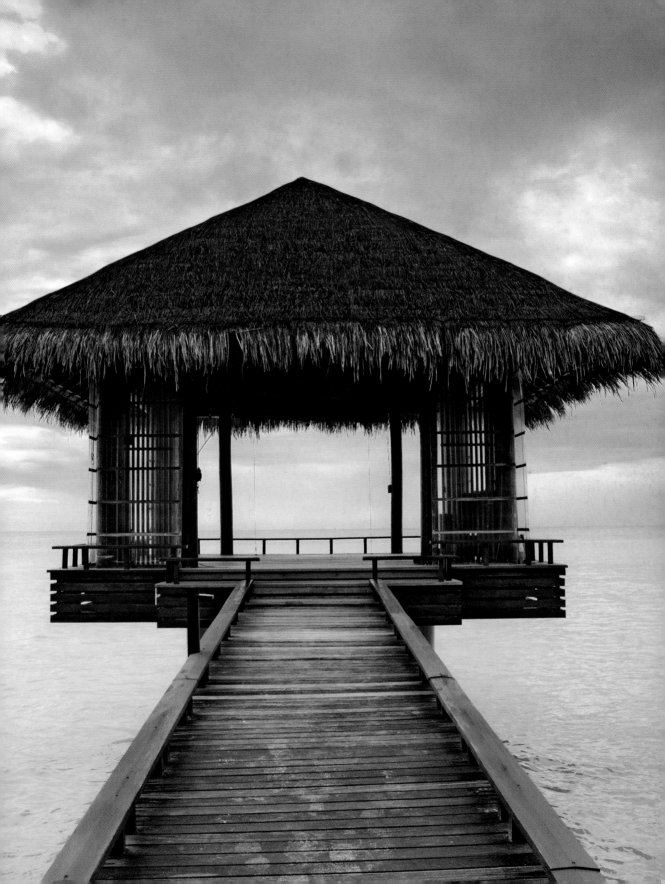

Most of us are stressed. Family, work, partners, children – no matter how much we love them, they usually cause us stress. Then there are the things that we don't love that cause us even more stress – money worries, work worries, difficult people, traffic jams. In modern life, it's pretty hard to escape stress, which is why, with the best will in the world, all my clients suffer from stress to a certain degree.

Now the bad news is, stress really doesn't help us win the battle of the tummy bulge. Studies show that the stress hormone cortisol (which we release when we're anxious) causes our bodies to dump fatty deposits all over our tummies and waists. It's an outdated defence mechanism from hundreds – even thousands – of years ago when we needed fat to keep us alive because we weren't always sure where our next meal was coming from. So, during times of stress (say, during a particularly cold winter, which could potentially lead to famine, or when we were at risk of attack from a wild animal), we needed extra fat reserves for warmth, and to keep us energised if we needed to go without food for a while or if we had to fight or run away from danger. Women in particular needed extra fat – especially around their tummies – for extra protection during pregnancy and breastfeeding.

Nowadays, however, a cold winter won't affect us (thanks to central heating), and we're unlikely to be short of food. We nearly always have enough to eat several times a day; and even if we don't, most of us have enough fat on our bodies to keep us going should we end up having to skip a meal or two. But Mother Nature doesn't know this, and when we get anxious and the stress hormone cortisol floods our body, she makes sure we have enough padding around our mid-section to deal with whatever stress is heading our way. So, although stressors nowadays are hopefully non-life-threatening (traffic jams or arguments with our partner, for example), and therefore completely different from those thousands of years ago, we're still going to get a build-up of fat around our waists and tummies in response. Being stressed all the time is literally like sticking an extra inch of fat on your tummy.

EAT YOURSELF LESS STRESSED

I can't advise my clients on how to deal with their stressful jobs, family lives or even the traffic jams that they encounter on their way to work every day. But what I can do is to help them reduce stress in a few other ways – firstly, by eating themselves less stressed.

The food we eat has a huge impact on our stress levels – some foods calm our bodies down, helping to lower levels of cortisol and reduce the amount of fat we lay down on our tummies. Other foods, however, do the opposite and cause our bodies to feel even more stressed, which increases cortisol levels and fat distribution.

Tummy-toning foods

All of the following foods reduce stress which, in turn, will keep your tummy nice and flat:

BLUEBERRIES

These are top of my list because they're a low GI (glycaemic index) food, which means they keep your blood-sugar (and energy) levels nice and steady. Eat a handful of blueberries every single day, if you can.

GREEN VEGETABLES

Broccoli, kale, asparagus – it doesn't matter which ones you go for – all green vegetables are packed with vitamins that help to replenish and soothe a stressed body. Remember: the darker the better (so, for example, dark green rocket contains more goodness than a pale green iceberg lettuce). Most green vegetables also contain potassium, which, according to studies, calms the nerves.

My two favourite green vegetables are spinach and broccoli. Just 30g of spinach gives you 40 per cent of your daily magnesium requirement (insufficient magnesium leads to headaches and fatigue). Broccoli is full of stress-relieving B vitamins; it also contains folic acid which can reduce feelings of stress and depression.

RED, YELLOW AND ORANGE VEGETABLES

These include tomatoes, carrots and peppers, which are rich in vitamins and minerals and are shown to lower stress levels. They also contain lots of fibre; this is helpful in treating both constipation and loose bowels, which are often caused by irritable bowel syndrome (IBS), one of the most common side effects of too much stress.

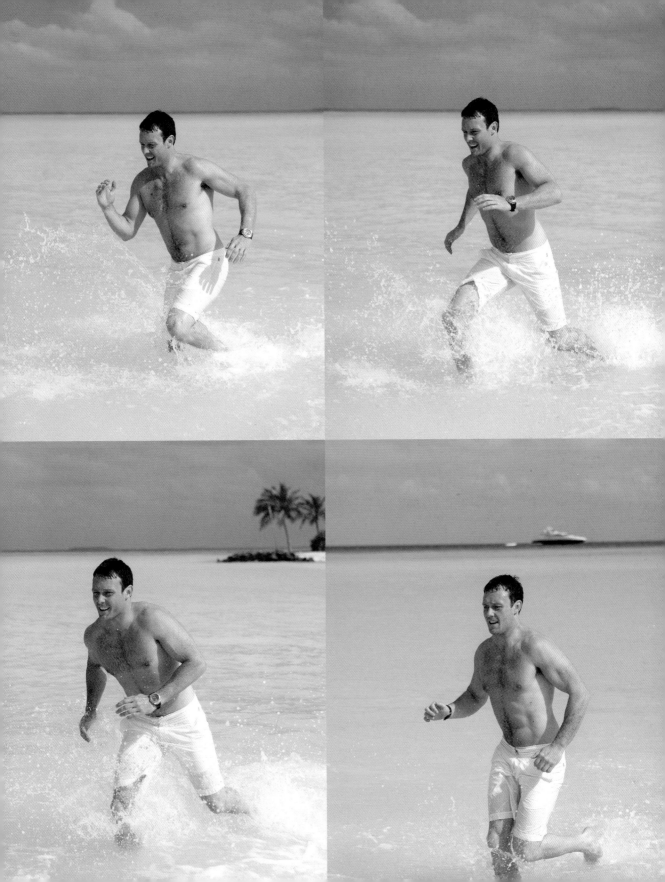

TURKEY

Turkey contains an amino acid called L-tryptophan, which triggers the release of serotonin (a relaxing feelgood brain chemical). Chicken is also high in this amino acid.

WATER

Even mild dehydration stresses your body out, so it's important to drink at least 2–3 litres of still, room-temperature water every single day. Sip it regularly throughout the day. Filtered is best; tap water is less good.

YOGURT

This provides a good hit of minerals, including calcium which is important for your nerves. Yogurt also neutralises the acidity caused by stress. Don't go for the low-fat stuff though (it's often packed full or sugar and sweeteners, which stress out your body) – choose a natural and organic one instead.

OILY FISH

Salmon, tuna and mackerel contain lots of Omega fatty acids which protect your heart (your heart can also get a battering from too much stress). Omega fatty acids also control levels of cortisol and adrenaline (another stress hormone) in the body, plus they contain choline, which is great for your improving memory and concentration. Limit your tuna intake to one fresh steak (or three tins) a week though, as it contains mercury, too much of which is bad for you.

CHOCOLATE

Chocolate acts as a mood elevator. It also contains magnesium which calms and soothes fragile nerves. The key here, however, is in the portion size: a little bit, like 1 or 2 squares, once or twice a week is OK; too much definitely isn't, however, because it's packed with sugar.

ALMONDS, PISTACHIOS AND WALNUTS

These are full of vitamins B and E, which boost your immune system (whereas stress weakens it). Plus, pistachios lower your blood pressure (whereas stress raises it). Have a small handful of nuts every day.

Does your stomach churn when you're stressed? Your digestive system starts working erratically or shuts down completely when you're anxious, which is why highly stressed people often get stomach ulcers. Stress impacts hugely on the health and appearance of your tummy, so if you want a flat stomach you really need to tackle your stress levels.

AVOCADOS

These help to lower blood pressure because of all the monounsaturated fat and potassium they contain. They have more potassium than bananas, according to several studies, plus they satisfy creamy/sweet cravings better.

CANTALOUPE MELON

This is an excellent source of vitamin C, which is great for beating stress.

BEEF

Beef is full of iron, zinc and B vitamins, all of which have been shown to chill you out. However, you should limit yourself to 1 or 2 portions a week.

Foods that stress your body out

The following foods can all put stress on your body and should be avoided or, at least, limited:

ALCOHOL

Alcohol is full of sugar, which ages you from the inside and stresses out your whole system.

CAFFEINE

In sensible doses, this is absolutely fine (say, 1 cup of regular coffee or up to 6 cups of green tea a day). However, any more than this puts your system on to 'high alert' and cortisol will flood your body (see p. 30) – which equals a fat tummy.

FIZZY DRINKS

Again, these are full of sugar, so should be cut out of your diet.

SALT

Commercial table salt stresses out your system and raises blood pressure. Go for organic sea salt instead, which is full of healthy minerals.

PROCESSED DAIRY FOODS

These include cheap cheeses, low-fat yogurts and so on. If they're heavily processed or full of sugar and sweeteners, they can cause inflammation in the gut.

PRESERVATIVES

As I explained in the previous chapter, your body doesn't know how to process the preservatives found in junk and processed foods. Just eat clean and lean foods.

TOO MUCH SUGAR

I've covered sugar in more detail on p. 15, but put simply, sugar causes enormous stress on the system – avoid it at all costs.

FOODS YOU'RE SENSITIVE TO

Wheat and gluten are the most common stress-causing allergens. They can really inflame the bowel, causing a swollen stomach just below the belly button. Go without them for a week and see if it makes a difference.

Wheat and gluten are found mainly in:

* Breads
* Most breakfast cereals
* Pasta
* Muffins
* Pastries
* Baked goods
* Pizza bases
* Pie crusts
* Biscuits
* Cakes
* Croissants
* Bagels
* Alcohol made from grains – i.e. beer, whisky, bourbon and liqueurs
* Cheese spreads
* Couscous
* Tomato ketchup
* Processed meats
* Margarines
* Oats
* Salad dressings
* Sausages
* Seasoning mixes
* Semolina
* Soy sauce and most Chinese sauces
* Sweets which contain grain (stabilisers made from gluten)
* Tinned meats containing preservatives

Eating habits that stress your body out

As well as what you eat, the way you eat can also affect your stress levels:

YO-YO DIETING

Constantly swinging between starving yourself on a fad diet, then gorging yourself when you can't keep it up any longer, wreaks havoc with your blood-sugar levels and digestion. Just take it easy and keep your eating clean, lean and steady. The weight will then fall off – and stay off.

LONG PERIODS BETWEEN MEALS

If you go for more than 4 or 5 hours without eating anything, your body starts to think that it's being starved, so cortisol floods your system to prepare for what it thinks is a famine. Plus, when you do finally eat, you're more likely to overeat or pick the wrong things because you're so hungry.

SKIPPING BREAKFAST

Always eat within an hour of waking up, otherwise your body will become stressed (see above). If you don't have time for breakfast, just grab a piece of fruit and a few nuts. Never, ever leave it longer than an hour.

DRINKING AT MEALTIMES

Drinking at mealtimes slows down your digestion, which can lead to bloating and gas. Always drink at least 15 minutes before or after eating a meal, but not during it. (It's OK – though not ideal – to drink with small snacks.)

EATING TOO QUICKLY

For optimum digestion, you must eat every mouthful slowly, chewing it at least 20 times. Don't eat when you're stressed, rushed or anxious, otherwise you'll stress out your digestion, which causes bloating. If you want a flat tummy, take it slowly and relax while you eat.

NOT DRINKING ENOUGH WATER

Dehydration is very stressful to the body. Drink at least 2–3 litres of still, filtered water a day. Put a slice of lemon in your first glass of the day to make your body even cleaner.

KICK-STARTING YOUR DAY WITH CAFFEINE

One cup of coffee is OK in the morning, but only drink it after you've eaten most of your breakfast. Never drink coffee on an empty stomach.

NOT EATING ENOUGH FIBRE

Insufficient fibre leads to stress and inflammation of the bowels, and this makes your tummy look bigger.

EXERCISE YOURSELF LESS STRESSED

Exercise smarter, not harder, is something I say a lot to my clients. If you're trying to achieve that flat tummy fast, don't go mad with too much exercise. Be smart about it, and get more out of less exercise.

The following three exercises reduce cortisol levels in the body, helping you to achieve a flat tummy. They help to unblock and move energy through the body and target stubborn tummy fat. Plus, they help to regulate breathing patterns. All of which helps the abdominals stay strong and flat. If you do these exercises before bed, they'll set you up for 8 hours of optimal fat-burning sleep (in the next chapter, I explain why sleeping keeps you slim). Think about your breathing; inhaling through the nose and exhaling through the mouth, and the slower and more controlled the moves are, the better.

Breathing squat

I want you to go as slow and as low as possible here. This exercise will help to focus you on a controlled breathing pattern and to increase flexibility in your hips.

✳ Take a comfortable stance with your feet shoulder-width apart and your arms held out in front of you parallel to the floor.

✳ Inhale through your nose, then lower yourself down as far as you can comfortably go as you exhale.

✳ Pause for a few seconds, then inhale as you return to standing.

✳ Try to focus on lowering for a 3-second pause.

✳ Repeat 10 times.

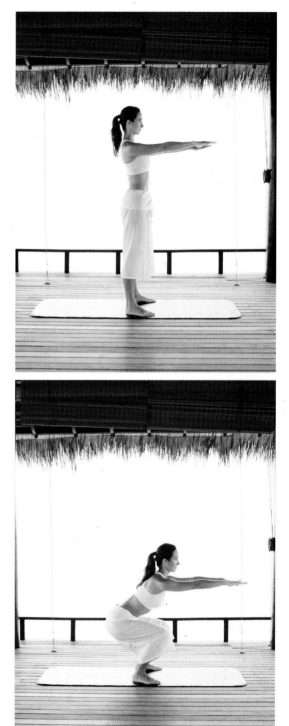

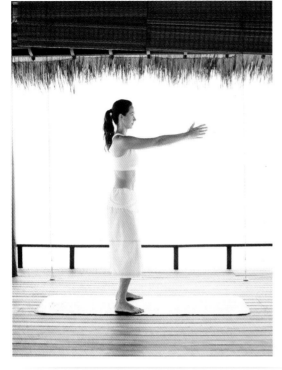

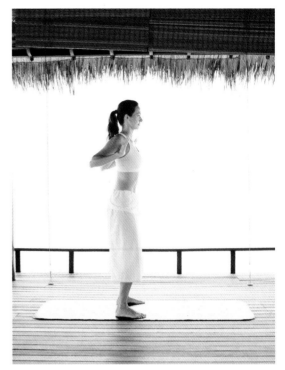

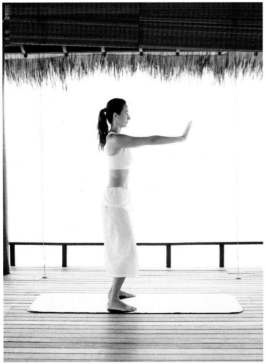

Energy push

This exercise helps to improve digestion.

✳ Take a comfortable stance with your feet shoulder-width apart and your arms held out in front of you with your palms facing each other.

✳ Inhale and bring your hands back in towards your body.

✳ Exhale and push your arms out back to start position.

✳ Repeat 20 times, focusing on slow breathing.

*quick fix
These movements can be done whenever you need to relax or wind down.

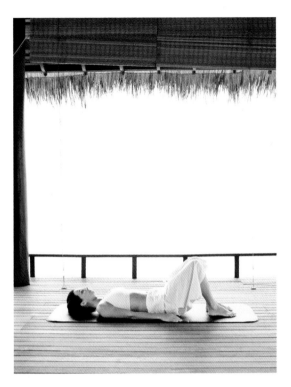
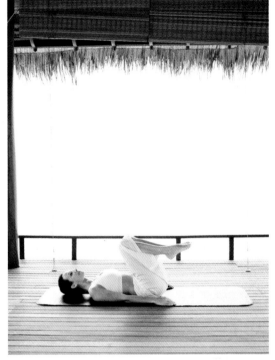

Leg tuck

This is great for the lower abdominals. It's a very important exercise in that it helps with energy blockage in people who are having problems with relationship stress from partners or family. Moving the legs towards the chest helps to strengthen up the abdominals, but also brings energy into the pelvis.

* Lie on your back with your feet on the floor, and your knees bent.

* Inhale, then bring your legs into your chest as you exhale.

* Inhale again, as you return your legs to the floor. Try to establish a natural breathing pattern.

* Repeat 10 times.

Note: if you get back pain while doing this exercise, place a small towel under your lower back and gently draw your belly towards your spine when you inhale.

Breathe better. One of the most efficient ways of controlling your stress levels is to make sure you're breathing correctly. Shallow breathing (which we do automatically when we're stressed) causes an increase in the stress hormone, cortisol. Proper breathing – whereby your belly inflates and, as you slowly exhale, you feel calm – really reduces stress. No matter what situation you're in, you're just one breath away from reducing your stress levels – and making your tummy flat!

HAVE A STRESS DETOX!

Here's how:

✶ Limit the amount of time you spend watching TV or browsing on your computer. So many of my clients admit to coming home from work, switching on their TV and then surfing websites on their laptops. This will suck the life out of you, disrupt your sleep and overstimulate your brain. Only watch 1 or 2 TV shows that you like, or go online to do something specific – never both at the same time, and not for longer than an hour or two, maximum, per evening.

✶ Stay away from 'energy vampires'. You know the ones I'm talking about – 'friends', colleagues or family members who drain you of energy with their negative attitude. Family members are harder to avoid (especially close ones, like mothers!). In all seriousness, be careful of people who take the wind out of your sails.

✶ Sort through your emotions. If you're prone to depression and anxiety, or unhappy in your job or relationship, then do something about it. Don't go through life feeling unhappy. Go for some counselling, break up with the person who's making you unhappy or change your job (again, where possible).

✶ Laugh a lot. It sounds cheesy, but spend time with people who make you laugh or do things that you find fun.

✶ Have a massage. Do this every week if you can afford it, as it releases calming, feelgood hormones into the body. If you can't afford it, get your partner or a friend to give you a foot or shoulder rub!

✶ Have some down time every day. Whether you're alone, or with your favourite person, spend at least 30 minutes of every day doing something relaxing.

✶ Sort out your finances. Nothing makes you more stressed than unopened bills or mounting debts. File your paperwork, and speak to experts about sorting out your debts if you have any.

✶ Avoid unreasonable to-do lists. This applies especially to women. There are no medals for an immaculate house or a packed social calendar. Stop giving yourself so many things to do (unless, of course, you're the kind of person who thrives on being busy).

✶ Approach things, including this programme, with a positive way of thinking. Your life is shaped by what you 'feed' yourself physically, emotionally and spiritually.

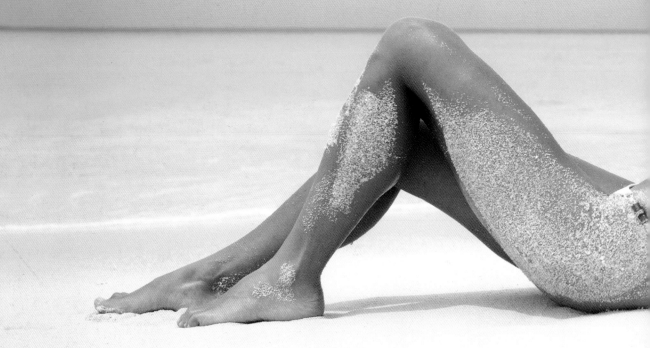

STRESS-BUSTING MINERALS AND HERBS

The following are great for stress-busting and should feature strongly in your clean & lean diet:

MINERALS

✳ **Magnesium** – a natural mood stabiliser and calming agent, it's found naturally in spinach and pumpkin.

✳ **Potassium** – this helps to prevent high blood pressure and, therefore, stress; the best natural sources are potatoes, avocados, fish, chicken, leeks and bananas.

✳ **Iron** – low levels weaken the body's ability to deal with stress; it can be found naturally in peas, red meat, eggs and potatoes.

HERBS

✳ **Camomile** – a great anti-stress remedy, this also counteracts the effects of overindulging in fatty foods and alcohol.

✳ **Lavender** – helps you to relax and induces sleep, which is why it's often used in pre-bedtime rituals (lavender spray on pillows and so on).

✳ **Kava kava** – helps to reduce feelings of anxiety and depression.

✳ **Red clover** – this is shown to lower cholesterol and it reduces feelings of anxiety.

✳ **Rosemary** – improves blood flow to the muscles (which will help to relax them).

✳ **Sage** – studies show that this enhances memory and concentration (stress often lowers levels of concentration).

✳ **St John's wort** – a famous anti-depressant herb, this helps to lower levels of stress hormones in the body.

✳ **Dill** – this is great for digestive disorders, including indigestion, bloating, gas and irritable bowel syndrome (IBS), common in stressed people.

✳ **Tarragon** – this promotes a feeling of calm, and is known as 'nature's tranquilliser'.

✳ **Liquorice root** – this enables the body to deal with stress more efficiently, plus it keeps your blood-sugar levels steady (stress, as we've seen, can cause these to rise and fall rapidly).

✳ **Passion flower** – for years, this has been used to treat anxiety and insomnia.

CHAPTER 4

WHY SLEEP MAKES YOUR TUMMY FLAT

THIS CHAPTER WILL HELP YOU TO:

1. SLEEP YOURSELF SLIM
2. UNDERSTAND THE FOOD-SLEEP CONNECTION
3. REDUCE SUGAR CRAVINGS WITH SLEEP
4. IMPROVE YOUR SLEEP ROUTINE

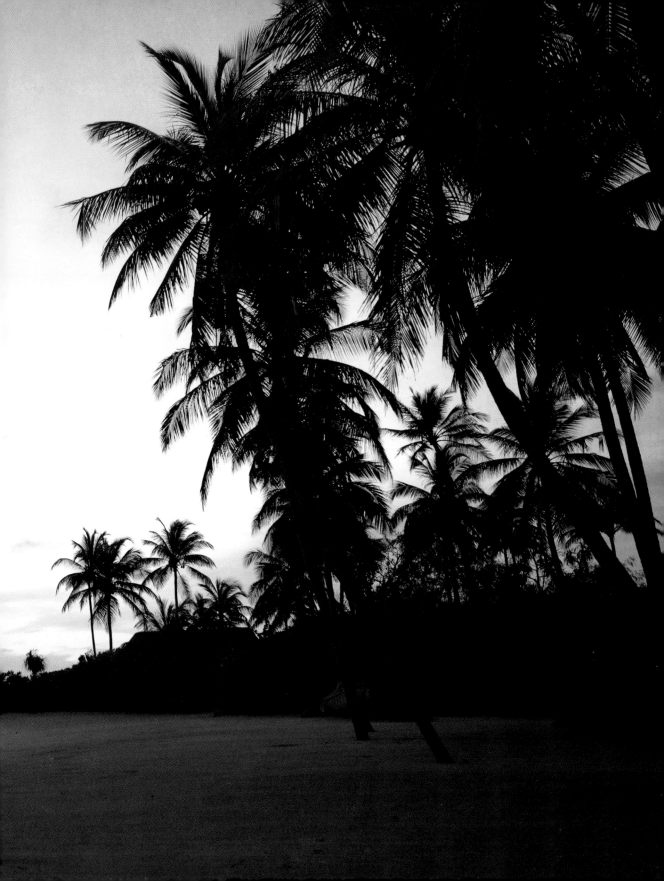

We've come a long way since going to bed when the sun sets and waking up when it rises. But this is how our bodies were – and still are – designed to function.

Nowadays, however, most of us sleep to a completely different timetable from our ancestors', and the one our body truly craves. I know I do. We wake up 'artificially' with the help of an alarm clock. Then we go to bed at, say, midnight, after keeping ourselves awake beforehand with more of what I call 'sleep vampires' (bright lights, TV, laptops and other stimulants like glasses of wine, sugary foods and cups of tea). Yet our bodies still crave our ancestors' simple, calming sleep patterns of going to bed when it gets dark outside, and waking up naturally when it gets light.

But what does all this have to do with weight loss and keeping your tummy flat? Well, quite simply, if you return to this old-fashioned way of sleeping, you'll lose weight – especially around your tummy and waist. Our modern lifestyle, with its accompanying sleep pattern, puts extra stress on the body, and as we learnt from the previous chapter, this is bad news for your waistline. The old way of sleeping, on the other hand, balances out fat-burning hormones and reduces stress and levels of cortisol (the stress hormone, which makes your body cling to fat around your middle). Another hormone called leptin is responsible for telling your brain when your stomach is full, and it also helps to control appetite and metabolism. Not sleeping properly disrupts this hormone, which is why you find yourself eating more when you're sleep deprived.

However, in the modern world it's practically impossible to stick to this outdated sleep schedule – especially if you have children, a job and other commitments. Neither do you have to go completely without sleep vampires. But there are ways of tweaking your sleep so it resembles our ancestors' schedule, but is practical for your life too.

HOW TO SLEEP YOURSELF SLIM

Let's look at some ways to help you sleep yourself slim:

IMPOSE AN 'ELECTRONIC SUNDOWN'

I tell my clients to turn off as many electronic items as possible in the lead-up to bedtime – all of these disrupt sleep by exciting your brain. That means in the hour or two before bed, you should turn off your laptop, TV and mobile phone, and stop texting and answering or making calls. Keep your lights low (use a low-wattage lamp or a dimmer switch). You need to make your environment dull and calm, in keeping with your natural body clock. Our ancestors didn't have TVs to keep them awake, so they drifted off to sleep much quicker than we do.

Be aware of the temperature in your bedroom. If it's too hot or too cold you won't sleep; the ideal is 16–18°C. If you're a really bad sleeper, buy a thermometer and check the temperature in your room – you may just discover that this is the reason for your inability to get a good night's sleep.

CHECK YOUR WINDOWS

If you have allergies, such as hay fever, make sure your windows are closed during the pollen season.

SLEEP WITH THE SEASONS

In the winter we need more sleep due to our internal body clock. As a rough guide, shorter, darker days (winter) mean we need more sleep, while longer, lighter days (summer) mean we can get by on less sleep.

TAKE POWER NAPS

If possible, have 15-minute power naps during the day. If you can't fall asleep, just have 15-minute lie-downs with no electronic gadgets, books or magazines. Just lie down with your eyes closed and breathe deeply. Even if you don't fall asleep, it will calm you down (reducing cortisol levels) and if you keep doing it at the same time every day (say, when you come home from work or weekend afternoons), eventually you will be able to drop off. Just don't have your phone in the room with you and keep your hands off the TV remote!

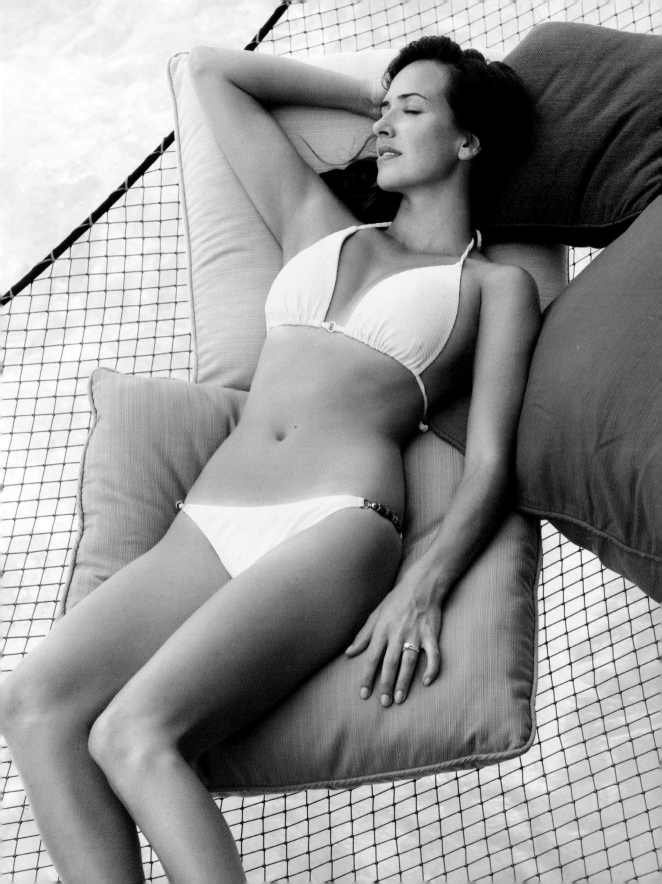

TRY BI-NEURAL BEATS

These were discovered by Heinrich Wilhelm Dove, a Prussian physicist, in 1839. He discovered that these beats influence and encourage the brain to fall asleep. You can download the sounds on to your iPhone or iPod, or you can buy bi-neural CDs.

USE BLACKOUT BLINDS OR AN EYE MASK

A blackout blind is a simple lining (it doesn't have to be black – they come in white and cream too) that doesn't let any sunlight, street lights or lights from passing traffic into your bedroom. Remember, your sleep environment (and pre-bed environment) needs to be as dark and as dull as possible to best aid sleep.

Failing that, buy an eye mask and pop it on just before you go to sleep.

AVOID CONFRONTATIONS BEFORE BED

If you're annoyed with your partner or children about something, write it down on a notepad next to your bed, and promise yourself you'll deal with it in the morning. Don't think about it at bedtime – just remember it's written down and you'll focus on it tomorrow.

ESTABLISH A BEDTIME ROUTINE

Anyone who has had a baby knows the importance of routine when it comes to getting babies sleeping through the night. The same goes for adults too. I recommend that my clients do something relaxing every night before bed – whether it's a bath, listening to music or reading a chapter of their favourite book – then go to sleep at the same time (give or take 30 minutes).

LISTEN TO CLASSICAL MUSIC IN THE EVENING

Studies show that classical music calms the brain. Listening to it during dinner will also slow down your eating, which means you'll get fuller quicker which, in turn, means you're likely to eat less.

DO SOME STRETCHING JUST BEFORE BED

Stretching will help to lower your cortisol levels, and release any tension from the day. I also tell my clients to squeeze every muscle from their head to their toe, while they're lying in bed. It sounds strange, but it really works: squeeze your eyes shut, screw up your face, bring your shoulders up to your ears, clench your fists and so on. This is also a good one to try if you have trouble napping during the day.

EAT MAGNESIUM-RICH FOODS

Such as broccoli, spinach, nuts and whole grains as these help the body to sleep. Or try my Body Serenity (available at www.bodyism.com).

HAVE SEX!

Having sex causes the release of endorphins into the body, which calms you down and induces sleep.

SLEEP AND THE NEW MUM

I train plenty of new mums, and many of them have trouble zipping up their knee-high boots all the way to the top, despite losing most of their baby weight. Anecdotely, it seems fatty deposits on the legs is typical for mums of newborns who have to get up several times in the night as sleep deprivation can result in low levels of the growth hormone which is predominantly released during sleep. If you are a new mum, try to get as much rest as you can. Daytime naps (when your baby is asleep), blackout blinds and stretching before bed will reduce your stress levels, restore your sleep hormones and boost fat burning. (And if you're not a new mum, sleeping better will still help you to lose fat from your legs!)

*case study

Erin came to see me complaining about her energy levels, and also the increase of fat around her belly button. Her diet was fairly balanced, but she told me she was averaging just 4 or 5 hours of sleep a night. She said she usually watched TV late into the evening, went to bed late and would often wake up more tired than when she went to bed. She worked as a school teacher, specifically with children who have learning difficulties. She also ran every morning, played field hockey at night, and on top of all this was renovating her house. After chatting with her, I realised her stress levels were very high. One of the first things I did was to tackle these because I realised they were impacting on her sleep. All the cardio she was dong was raising her cortisol levels, and she spent so much time working there was not enough time for resting and letting her body recover. Her sleep was poor as a result. Her adrenal glands were working overtime and she had adrenal fatigue.

I got Erin to reduce the time she spent exercising and implemented some power naps at lunchtime and on weekends. I also made sure she had a sleep routine whereby she would spend 10 minutes stretching before bedtime (which was now at the same time every evening) and I also told her to have a weekly massage. Her body quickly responded and her tummy fat disappeared in about 6 weeks, even though she hardly made any changes to her diet.

THE FOOD-SLEEP CONNECTION

How you sleep impacts hugely on your appetite and the foods you choose. So, after a good night's sleep, your body is happy with (and craves) clean and lean food – that's good-quality protein, dark green vegetables, oily fish, nuts, seeds, oils and berries. After a night of poor, broken or not enough sleep, your body becomes hungrier and craves sugar, fat and caffeine. Why? Because these quickly (albeit briefly) prop up your energy levels. That's why you feel like eating a sugary croissant with coffee when you're hungover, if you're a new mum or if you've had to get up early to go to the airport, for example. However, your blood-sugar levels will then drop rapidly, leaving you feeling hungrier and more tired than before. All the extra sugar will lay more fat on your tummy and love-handle area, project you into a very damaging cycle of jittery highs and crashing lows, give you a serious sugar-for-energy addiction and cause poor quality of sleep.

EAT YOURSELF SLEEPY

✳ Avoid caffeine for at least 6 hours before you go to bed – caffeine's mainly found in coffee, tea, green tea and chocolate. I'm a huge fan of green tea (it's packed with antioxidants and helps your body to burn fat), but I tell my clients to only drink it in the morning and afternoon – never later than 5 p.m.

✳ Avoid alcohol before bed – people think that alcohol is a relaxant. It isn't, it's a depressant – it will just give you a huge hit of sugar at the time when you should be winding down. Plus, it's dehydrating, meaning you'll probably wake up thirsty for water in the middle of the night. And if you don't, you'll wake up with a headache and a dry mouth.

✳ Eat foods that are rich in tryptophan – studies show that if you eat these during the day, you'll sleep better that night. Tryptophan-rich foods include nuts, beans, fish and eggs, so try to tuck into at least 1 of these every day.

✳ Eat serotonin-releasing foods – studies also show that certain foods release serotonin (the feelgood hormone) into our bodies, making us sleepier; these include turkey, milk and bananas.

HOW SUGAR IMPACTS ON SLEEP

The biggest sleep vampire of all is sugar, which is why I'm devoting a whole section to it here, although it's already been mentioned previously. You will have learnt in Chapters 1 and 2 that you can never be clean and lean if you regularly eat sugar because it's a horrid, fattening toxin that makes you fat and wrinkly. But it also makes you sleep deprived because, as we've seen, it causes your blood-sugar levels to rise too rapidly. It also causes you to wake up hungry for more sugar and other fattening foods.

When you're tired – for whatever reason – the temptation is to 'eat yourself awake' and sugar is nearly always the first thing you reach for. However, if you want a decent night's sleep, you need to take sugar off the menu and stick to the clean and lean, sleep-inducing foods I've already mentioned instead. Avoid the following at least 6 hours before bedtime (of course, you should be avoiding them altogether if you want to be truly clean and lean):

✳ White refined sugar
✳ Fruit juices
✳ White, non-organic pasta, bread and rice
✳ Alcohol (it's literally all sugar)
✳ Cakes, sweets, biscuits and ice cream
✳ Low-fat foods, such as diet yogurts, most processed breakfast cereals, health bars, muffins and energy drinks
✳ Anything that contains an ingredient ending in '-ose' (sucrose, glucose, maltose, lactose, dextrose and fructose); these are basically another word for sugar
✳ Anything containing high-fructose corn syrup; again, this is sugar by another name
✳ All sweeteners

*case study

Eva had a great approach to diet and exercise. She did aerobics a couple of times a week, Pilates at the weekend and ate lots of clean and lean foods with only a few treats. However, she had a stubborn bit of fat on her tummy that she just couldn't shift. Having established that her diet and exercise routines were both good, I asked her about her stress levels, which were low. Then we discussed her sleeping habits and Eva revealed that she was a bit of an insomniac and her sleeping routine was very erratic. I told her she would need to tweak her sleeping habits if she ever wanted to say goodbye to that little bit of fat on her tummy.

Eva's bedroom was on a busy street, meaning that her room was never fully dark, so the first thing I told her was to have her curtains fitted with a blackout lining. Next, I told her to impose a 9 p.m. 'electronic shutdown' (the only thing she could keep on was her lamp). She found this tough because she was used to texting and emailing late into the evening, often in bed (no wonder she couldn't sleep!). I also suggested that she take a bath before bed with a few drops of lavender oil. And, with just these few tiny tweaks, Eva lost that little bit of tummy fat.

CHAPTER 5

WHAT KIND OF TUMMY DO YOU HAVE?

THIS CHAPTER WILL HELP YOU TO:

1. DISCOVER WHAT TYPE OF TUMMY YOU HAVE

2. LEARN NEW WAYS TO KEEP IT FLAT

3. WORK OUT HOW TO HAVE A FLAT TUMMY AT ANY AGE

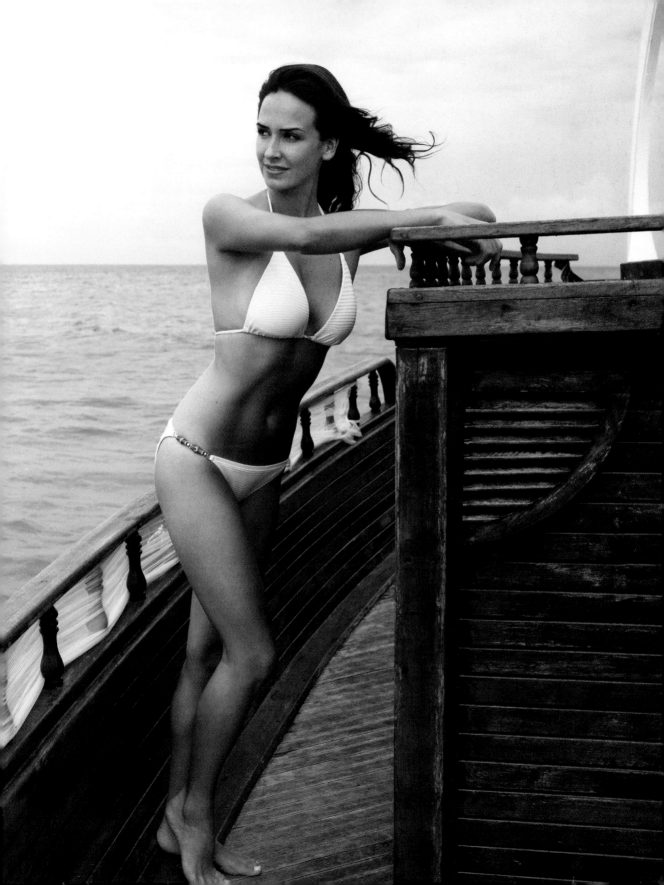

Now, just as women's bums, breasts, legs and arms all have different shapes, there are also lots of tummy shapes out there. And I've seen them all. Most of my female clients – even the models – moan about their stomachs and I've spent years working out clever ways of sculpting and flattening them. But to do that, I needed to know what kind of tummy they had.

Less-than-flat tummies can be caused (partly) by genetics and your natural body shape. For example, women who are slim but have big hips and thighs tend to have very flat stomachs (these women probably refer to themselves as 'pear shaped'), whereas women with very slim legs and narrow hips often carry their weight around their stomachs (these women are often known as 'apple shaped'). However, the most likely cause of a flabby stomach is the wrong type of food, drink, lifestyle and even posture. A woman with bad posture and an addiction to fizzy drinks is more likely to have a fatter, more pronounced stomach than one who has great posture and only drinks water.

THE DIFFERENT TUMMY TYPES – WHICH DO YOU HAVE?

If you can identify your stomach type from the following descriptions, then I can highlight where you're (probably) going wrong and, more importantly, what you can do about it. You may fall into a couple of categories, which is very common – in this case, follow the instructions for the one you identify most strongly with, then take some pointers from any others which also relate to you and combine the advice.

The post-baby tummy

You'll know if you have this type, simply because you've had children and have a little tummy as a result.

After giving birth, your uterus is around 15 times heavier than it was pre-pregnancy. It then takes approximately 6 weeks to return to its previous size and weight, so don't even think about getting a flat stomach before then. Allow your body to heal and rejuvenate in good time.

However, a few months – or even years – after childbirth, a lot of my clients want to do something about their 'mummy tummy' – the term they use to describe their stomach – which may be slightly flabbier, looser or more wobbly than it was pre-baby. The good news is, the remedy isn't hundreds of sit-ups every day and a strict diet. Instead, the first thing I tell them to do is gentle pelvic-floor exercises. These act as a natural corset for the body and tighten you up from the inside out, resulting in a flatter stomach.

Your pelvic-floor muscles are the ones you would use if you were trying to stop yourself from peeing. Squeeze and clench them (as if you're stopping the flow) up to 15 times. You may need to work up to this number. Do 15 to 20 squeezes, 5 times a day. You can do them anywhere, and nobody will even know you're doing them. However, don't do them when you're on the toilet and actually 'mid-flow', as this can cause infection and stop your bladder from emptying properly. Instead, do them when you're at your desk at work or doing your make-up. As a way of remembering to do them, I tell my clients to pick 5 times a day when they're standing still and always to do their repetitions then.

Diet-wise, my biggest recommendation for women with a 'mummy tummy' is fish oil supplements as they turn on their fat-burning hormones and – crucially – switch off their fat-storing hormones. To start with, take 3 capsules every day – 1 with each main meal. Eventually, build up to 5 capsules a day. Elle Macpherson takes her fish oil supplements every day, and her stomach definitely thanks her for it!

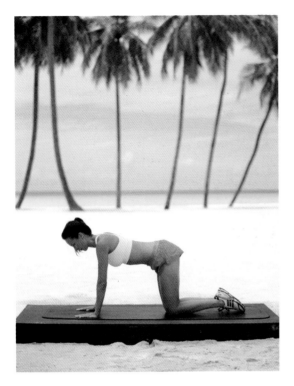

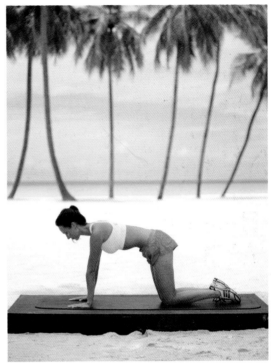

The best post-baby tummy exercise

This is one of the best exercises for getting your abs stronger again, plus it stops post-pregnancy incontinence (having a baby puts enormous pressure on your pelvic-floor muscles). It will also help keep your back strong, making it safer when lifting your little angel! It really works your lower abdominals, which are a very important muscle group as they help to stabilise the lower back and hips. This exercise is great for women who have had both a natural birth or a C-section. However, it is important to speak to your GP at your 6-week check-up before attempting any of these exercises.

The stomach vaccum

✳ Start on all fours, with your back straight and your arms slightly bent at the elbows. Your ears should be in alignment with your shoulders and hips.

✳ Relax your abdominals and take a big breath from the belly so it expands towards the floor.

✳ Slowly exhale and draw your belly button towards your spine, at the same time doing a pelvic-floor exercise. Your back should remain straight at all times.

✳ Once the air is completely gone, hold your belly towards your spine for 5 seconds.

✳ Repeat the process 20 times.

*it's easy!

When we say 'set the core' we mean to draw the belly gently towards the spine – not a full, harsh suck-in, just a gentle pull.

The bloated tummy

This kind of stomach is very common. I see it on lots of slim women, who have great arms and legs but a swollen, distended, bloated stomach. It's nearly always caused by inflammation of their digestive organs – usually the small intestine or colon. Swelling typically occurs in the lower part of their stomach (the bit below the belly button) and no amount of sit-ups or dieting will shift it. Does this sound familiar?

Inflammation is usually caused by food intolerances and allergies or sluggish bowels (or a combination or both).

FOOD INTOLERANCE AND ALLERGIES

To discover if you have an intolerance or allergy, you need to identify the foods you react to and cut them out for a week or two and see if this makes a difference to your stomach. Everybody has different intolerances, but the most common ones that I see are to wheat, gluten, alcohol, yeast and processed dairy. Eliminate foods 1 at a time, and reintroduce them 2 weeks later to see if they make a difference to your stomach (not just its size and appearance, but also how much gas, indigestion and discomfort you have).

Wheat and gluten are typically found in:
* Bread and pasta (unless otherwise stated)
* Most breakfast cereals
* Muffins
* Pastries
* Baked goods
* Pizza bases
* Pie crusts
* Biscuits
* Cakes
* Croissants
* Bagels
* Alcohol made from grains – i.e. beer, whisky, bourbon and liqueurs
* Cheese spreads
* Tomato ketchup
* Processed meats
* Margarine
* Oats
* Salad dressings
* Sausages
* Seasoning mixes
* Semolina
* Soups (apart from homemade)
* Soy sauce and most Chinese sauces
* Sweets which contain grain (stabilisers made from gluten)

Alcohol is typically found in:
* Beer
* Wine
* Alcopops
* Cocktails
* White spirits (vodka, gin, etc.)
* Alcohol made from grains – i.e. whisky, bourbon and liqueurs

Yeast is found in:
* Most breads (unless otherwise stated)
* Croissants
* Pastries
* Doughnuts
* Crumpets
* Muffins
* Beer and cider
* Marmite – and other yeast extracts such as Vegemite, stock cubes, gravy granules, etc.
* Vinegars

Processed dairy foods include:
* Cheese
* Milk
* Yogurt
* Cream
* Butter
* Ice cream

For a comprehensive list, visit bodyism.com.

SLUGGISH BOWELS

Another possible reason for a bloated stomach is an inflamed or sluggish bowel. This happens when you eat the wrong types of food and in the wrong way. Here's the wrong – and right – way to treat your bowels:

● Eating too quickly and not chewing properly: this irritates your bowels, and can cause poorly chewed and undigested food to sit and ferment in the gut (which then leads to bloating).
Instead: eat in a relaxed, calm environment. Never eat when you're stressed – if you're busy, simply wait until you can devote at least 20 minutes to a meal. And chew each mouthful at least 20 times – more if you can.
● Not drinking enough water: dehydration causes fluid retention, which causes bloating.
Instead: drink around 2–3 litres of still, filtered water every single day without fail. However, don't drink too close to mealtimes as this will disrupt the digestion of food and cause more bloating. As a general rule, try not to drink anything for 15 minutes before and after eating. And don't gulp down huge amounts too quickly (you'll swallow air,

which causes bloating too). Take small, regular sips throughout the day instead.
● Eating too many acidic foods: read Chapter 2 to remind yourself why acidic foods cause bloating.
Instead: eat more alkaline foods (see Chapter 2 for a reminder of what these are). Aim to make 70–75 per cent of everything you eat alkaline, and the rest acidic.
● Eating late at night: your digestion is at its peak at the beginning of the day and slows down after that. Remember, badly digested food sits in the gut and causes bloating.
Instead: make breakfast your biggest meal of the day and avoid food just before bedtime. It's a myth that eating late at night makes you gain more weight, but it does cause bloating, which ultimately makes it look as though you've gained weight.

The stress tummy

The stress tummy is very easy to identify. The bloating is normally quite distinct, with comparatively little body fat on the arms, legs and even the back. Physically, this belly is usually fairly hard unlike the soft, wobbly fat of an 'overweight tummy' (see opposite). Another big giveaway is the personality type of the person carrying the 'stress tummy'. They're typically over-achievers, with a perfectionist streak, a long to-do list (be it for work or home) and they're normally highly stressed. They may also suffer from stress-related conditions such as irritable bowel syndrome (IBS), which makes their stomach look even worse than it actually is.

The first thing I tell clients with a stress tummy is to ditch the following:

* coffee/tea * soft drinks * processed foods
* drugs (legal and illegal) * alcohol
* tobacco * sugar

*reminder
Work with your body not against it.
Listen to what it is telling you.

. . . in favour of these stress-relieving alternatives:

● Camomile, ginger, chicory, cinnamon, lemon or peppermint tea

● Still, room-temperature filtered water with a slice of fresh lemon or lime (both are alkalising), peeled ginger, vanilla essence or fresh mint leaves

● Clean, lean, fresh, unprocessed foods (see Chapter 2 for a reminder of what these are)

● Fish oil supplements

● Magnesium-rich foods (magnesium is a calming mineral); these include dark green vegetables, almonds, Brazil nuts and sunflower seeds (see Chapter 2 for more examples of what to try)

● Bodyism's Body Serenity is my personal favourite (available at www.bodyism.com) – that's why I invented it!

You should also try to adopt the following lifestyle stress-relieving tips:

● Don't over-commit yourself

● Try to incorporate stress-busting habits into your day, such as long, warm baths, stretching, exercise and calming meditation

● Take as many holidays as you can afford – a relaxing week away takes fat off a stomach more effectively than any exercise programme ever could – I promise! After I'd explained this to one of my highly stressed clients he asked me, 'Is that why I lose so much weight when I go to the Greek Islands and drink a bottle of red wine every night and eat a big breakfast every morning?' And the answer is yes (even though he was consuming far more alcohol and calories than I would have liked – but I let that go) because his main source of stress (work) was out of the picture and that outweighed all the alcohol and fried food he was tucking into. Imagine how much more fat he would have dropped if he'd eaten well!

The overweight tummy

This is caused by carrying too much fat all over your body. Many overweight women tend to store a lot of their fat around their mid-section, and less, perhaps, on their legs and arms and other parts of the body.

Also known (rather cruelly) as a spare tyre, this type of stomach fat is the easiest to deal with. The fat is generally squidgy and soft, so is easier to remove than hard, toxic fat. It's often caused by a lack of exercise and too many calories, usually taken from alcohol, sugar, refined carbohydrates (biscuits, cakes, white bread and so on) and starchy carbohydrates (such as rice, bread and pasta).

To get rid of this type of tummy you need to stop eating these fat storers in the order that I've listed them. So give up 1) alcohol, then 2) sugar, then 3) refined carbs, then 4) starchy carbs. It's that simple. Then replace them all with clean and lean foods, such as whole protein (wild fish, organic eggs and organic non-processed meats) and non-starchy carbs (such as colourful vegetables).

The little 'pooch'

This is very similar to the bloated tummy, but is not as hard and swollen. I see a lot of very slim people with a little pooch tummy and it ruins their outline. It's nearly always the lower part of their stomach. There are several reasons for a pooch tummy, but the most common causes are an abdominal wall that's not working correctly, previous pregnancies or poor nutrition.

A MALFUNCTIONING ABDOMINAL WALL

This can be caused by doing the wrong type of abdominal exercise. The abdominals are like any other muscle group and if you do the wrong types of exercises you can weaken them. For example, I've noticed that very slim women who go to the gym a lot do lots of crunching exercises. If done excessively or incorrectly, this can place too much strain on the hip flexor muscles. In my experience, these women also tend to gravitate towards the 'gimmick' machines, such as ab rollers and ab-crunching machines. These are OK (albeit expensive) when used very carefully, but used badly or too much, they can cause an increase in your lower-back curve, which strains your hip flexors (the muscles that help keep your tummy flat). And it's this strain that can give you the pooch-belly look.

*reminder
Be kind to your body, breathe and stretch. They both help your body stay relaxed and energised.

So try instead the

Half-kneeling Lunge Stretch

(this loosens your hip flexors and can undo some of the damage done to a poor abdominal wall):

✳ Place one knee on the ground on a soft mat or pad with the arm on that side raised and the other leg bent in front, parallel to the floor.

✳ Keeping a slight forward lean of the torso, tighten your abs and squeeze your bottom on the side with the knee on the ground.

✳ Maintaining this posture, shift your entire body slightly forward.

✳ Exhale and hold the stretch for 3 seconds.

✳ Repeat 5 times on each leg.

PREVIOUS PREGNANCIES

When a woman has a Caesarean, her abdominal wall is cut and when it comes back to form it develops scar tissue where the incision was made. This scar tissue can interrupt the signals from the brain to the abdominal muscles, causing a delay in the brain telling the abdominals to brace themselves as you pick up something heavy. This delay can mean the abdominal muscles don't 'fire up', which places a strain on the lower-back muscles. (Your lower back often picks up the slack for lazy abs – hence why you can get lower-back pain when doing sit-ups incorrectly). This is easily resolved though with pelvic-floor exercises and properly executed lower-abdominal exercises.

However, even with a normal (vaginal) birth, women need to train their pelvic floor and lower abdominals, as this will help increase the blood flow to the abdominals (which will strengthen them).

POOR NUTRITION

An allergy to gluten can cause inflammation in the gut wall, leading to bloating and general discomfort in the lower abdominals (the bit below the belly button). This is where the pooch tummy is similar to the bloated tummy, so read the list of foods containing gluten on p. 54 and cut those foods out of your diet for a week or two to see if it makes a difference. If not, reintroduce them. If cutting them out does make your stomach flatter, the chances are your pot belly is due to an inflammation in the gut wall and you need to avoid gluten as much as possible.

Very hot chilli peppers can also cause irritation in your gut and, if you eat enough of them, this can cause your abdominal muscles to become weaker over time. Then there are the old favourites – sugar and refined carbs – which cause large deposits of fat to build up around your hips and tummy and won't help your pooch tummy either.

*reminder
Tune in to your body. See how the food you eat makes you feel.

*case study

Laura is a 57-year-old client of mine who has always loved hill walking. She's watched her weight all her life, and has always been in great shape. However, when she went through the menopause, no matter what she did, she had stubborn fatty deposits around her stomach, hips and thighs. HRT (Hormone Replacement Therapy) also changed her body shape and made her thicker around the middle. Because she had always been slim, it was incredibly frustrating for her that she could no longer control the weight around her tummy. Then she came to see me after a recommendation from a friend. I taught her all about my Clean & Lean approach, and I also taught her how to target her tummy fat. For a start, I told her to stop calorie counting and encouraged her to eat foods like avocados and nuts. Like a lot of people, she had always believed these types of foods to be fattening, until I told her that good fats actually helped your body to burn fat. Then I cut out all the sugar from her diet. This helped enormously, as despite her relatively good diet, she was a bit of a chocolate addict. By cutting out her daily dose of sugar, she no longer craved it because she was slowly becoming less toxic. After years of trying to keep her post-50 stomach flat with hill walking and various diets, the Clean & Lean approach stripped away that stubborn ring of fat in less than 2 months!

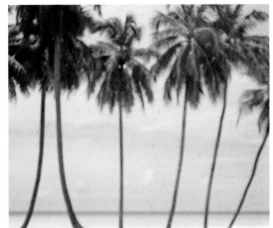

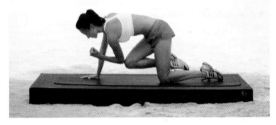

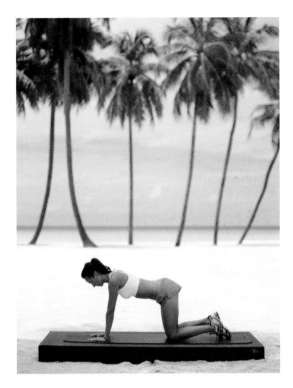

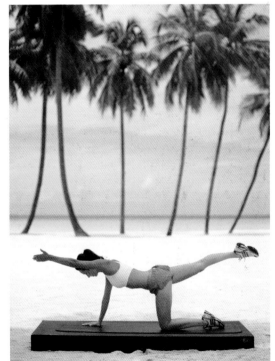

The four-point Superman exercise

Below is a brilliant post-baby tummy exercise.
Note: always wait until at least 6 weeks after giving
birth to exercise and always consult your doctor first.
✳ Start on all fours, with your back straight and your arms
slightly bent at the elbows. Your ears should be in
alignment with your shoulders and hips.

✳ Relax your abdominals and take a big breath from your
belly so that it expands. Breathe out, and once all the air is
expelled, lift your right hand and left knee off the floor.

✳ Bring your right elbow towards your stomach and your
left knee towards your chest so they both touch, keeping
your back straight at all times.

✳ Extend your right arm out in front of you at a 45-degree
angle and push your leg straight back, tensing the
opposite bottom cheek. Hold for 1 second.

✳ Return to the start position and swap sides.

✳ Perform 5–10 repetitions on each side.

HOW TO HAVE A FLAT TUMMY AT ANY AGE

My female clients range in age from 20-somethings to 50-somethings. When it comes to keeping their stomachs flat, I need to tweak their diet and exercise within the context of their age. That's not to say your stomach changes dramatically at the threshold of each decade, but each age group typically has to adopt a slightly different approach. Here are the general rules:

A 20-SOMETHING STOMACH

In your 20s, your body is close to its prime. You can get away with more (drinking alcohol, eating carbs, smoking, etc.) and your youth will soak it all up – for the most part. But if you overdo it, you will get fat – being a 20-something doesn't give you immunity against stomach fat. You can get great results at this age though, and for very little effort. The biggest thing to avoid is refined sugars (alcohol, sweets, biscuits, etc.) and complex carbohydrates (white bread, pasta, rice, etc.).

IDEAL EXERCISE

If you stay flexible, your abs will remain strong and your stomach flat, so try yoga or Pilates. Learn and practise good posture (if you haven't already) and keep your overall body fat down; this will keep your stomach flat with minimal effort.

*top tip
Good healthy habits are a choice that will last you a lifetime.

A 30-SOMETHING STOMACH

At this age you need to focus on the best choices because your metabolism starts to slow down a bit. Thirty-somethings need to eat mainly vegetable-based meals with a palm-sized serving of protein (such as chicken, fish, eggs or meat). Too many complex carbohydrates or refined sugars at this age (see p. 26 for examples) will cause an increase of insulin in the body, which will lead to an increase of fat around the sides. And fish oil supplements are a must – if you didn't take them in your 20s, definitely start taking them now (just to remind you, they help your body to burn fat around your middle).

IDEAL EXERCISE

Exercise-wise, people who have normally been very active in their 20s (either playing sport at university or going to the gym a lot when they're single or childless) tend to slow down as they reach their 30s. Because they have less free time thanks to a more demanding job perhaps, or a family, their activity levels often take a dip. Yet, crucially, their eating habits stay the same (or often deteriorate), which equals weight gain. This is just a general observation of some of my clients, and is not always the case. I also have clients who buck this trend and discover exercise in their 30s, having spent their 20s avoiding it.

Thirty-somethings should really vary their exercise – you need a mix of cardio (such as running, swimming, aerobics), weight training and flexibility (such as yoga or Pilates). Relaxing exercises are really important in your 30s, as your cortisol (the stress hormone) levels rise, causing belly fat. Regular massage (though not strictly an exercise!) is also a good habit to get into in your 30s, as it reduces cortisol build-up and stress.

A 40-SOMETHING STOMACH

Once you head into your 40s, your lean muscle mass starts to decrease. Quick reminder – you get lean muscle mass by eating the right foods and working out, and it makes you look firm and taut, and speeds up your metabolism. So what you eat now is even more important because the less lean muscle mass you have, the fewer calories you need.

Avoiding complex carbohydrates and refined sugar (yes, those two again) will help to reduce your insulin levels which, in turn, will help to slow down the amount of lean muscle mass you lose. You also need plenty of protein at this stage, as it provides the building blocks of lean muscle mass. Only eat red meat twice a week though, as it's harder to digest; the rest of the time stick to chicken, fish and eggs.

Fish oil supplements will help to regulate insulin levels and, at the same time, reduce inflammation. Whether from stress, too much caffeine or acidic foods, inflammation will cause fat to accumulate on your tummy and all over your body, so increasing your fish-oil consumption is an easy way of keeping your stomach as flat as possible post-40.

IDEAL EXERCISE

Strength training and flexibility exercises (such as Pilates) are very important at this age, as both increase lean muscle mass and will help to keep your stomach flat. The abdominals and pelvic-floor muscles need to be focused on now more than ever, so Pilates is the ideal choice – especially if you've had children. You should also take a daily fibre supplement, because your digestive system won't be as strong as it used to be.

A 50-SOMETHING STOMACH

This things you do in your 50s will work for you in your 70s, and 90s. Meals should be small, with as many coloured vegetables as possible, along with some lean protein. Red meat should only be eaten once a week. You need lots of calcium-rich foods to reduce your increased risk of the brittle-bone disease osteoporosis (see Chapter 2).

IDEAL EXERCISE

The majority should now be resistance based (using weights and pulleys) as this increases your lean muscle mass, as well as releasing serotonin (the feel-good hormone). It will also leave you with a strong core which will protect your hips, back and knees from injury, as well as keeping your stomach flat.

*case study

Charlotte came to us complaining about not being able to achieve a flat tummy (she also had an achy lower back). She'd had a natural birth with no complications a year before and exercised regularly. She had been seeing a personal trainer who focused entirely on core exercises, but she just wasn't seeing results. We discussed her eating habits and found that she loved spicy foods and had a cupcake each day at tea time (all that spice and sugar was weakening her abdominals).

One of the first things we did was to analyse her abdominals and we discovered that her pelvic floor and lower abdominals weren't working properly as a result of the birth – hence, the reason why all those sit-ups weren't working. We implemented a couple of breathing and pelvic-floor exercises, which we asked her to do 3 times a day. Her abdominals started to work immediately, so when we introduced core work her tummy really tightened up and became flatter. We also got her eating the Clean & Lean way, and stopped her from eating any gluten and spicy foods.

Within 10 weeks, Charlotte had regained her pre-pregnancy tummy – only even better than it was before.

BAD, BETTER AND BEST GUIDE TO A

BAD	BETTER	BEST
Bad: Croissants. **Why?** They're full of fat and sugar and very little goodness.	**Better:** Wholemeal bread with organic butter. **Why?** The fibre is good for digestion and the butter balances insulin levels.	**Best:** Gluten-free rice or spelt bread toasted with a quarter of an avocado. **Why?** No tummy-bloating gluten, plus a healthy serving of clean fat.
Bad: Pastries. **Why?** These are usually loaded with gluten and excess sugar which are your tummy's worst enemies.	**Better:** Wholemeal bread with a small serving of organic jam. **Why?** Organic jam is made without harmful pesticides and contains fewer preservatives.	**Best:** Organic yogurt with ¼ cup of mixed berries and a teaspoon of flaked almonds. **Why?** This is a perfect mix of carbs, protein and fats.
Bad: Doughnuts. **Why?** They're full of trans fats, gluten and sugar, and then on top of all that, they're deep-fried. This is the worst possible combination of ingredients and cooking methods – an evil little tummy fattener!	**Better:** Rice cakes with peanut butter. **Why?** Rice cakes are gluten-free and are easier to digest than other breads.	**Best:** Gluten-free bread with organic almond nut butter. Try various nut butters but make sure they're organic. **Why?** Nut butters are a great source of healthy fats. N.B. It's best to rotate nut butters in order to avoid an intolerance to 1 type of nut.
Bad: Crumpets. **Why?** They're a high-carbohydrate food containing all sorts of processed ingredients.	**Better:** Organic porridge made with organic milk or water. **Why?** Porridge is a low glycemic food, meaning it releases energy slowly over a long period of time.	**Best:** Gluten-free Irish soda bread with organic butter. **Why?** Irish soda bread is yeast-free and high in fibre.
Bad: Muffins. **Why?** Most high-street muffins have the same amount of sugar as cupcake icing. And forget the 'low-fat' ones. They're packed with sugar.	**Better:** An apple and a handful of nuts. **Why?** Fruit mixed with nuts is an excellent combination of proteins, carbohydrates and healthy fats.	**Best:** ¼ cup of gluten- and sugar-free muesli mixed with organic yogurt. **Why?** The muesli is a great source of carbohydrates and the yogurt is packed full of vitamins and minerals.
Bad: Beer and cider. **Why?** Both contain high amounts of sugar and are packed with calories.	**Better:** Organic cider or a light beer. **Why?** They have (slightly) less calories and alcohol.	**Best:** High-quality red wine. **Why?** The grape skins ar packed with resveratrol; a great antioxidant.
Bad: Stock cubes. **Why?** They're very high in salt.	**Better:** Reduced-salt organic stock cubes. **Why?** Less salt and preservatives.	**Best:** Homemade stock. **Why?** Even less salt and preservatives.

FLAT TUMMY AT ANY AGE

BAD	BETTER	BEST
Bad: Most vinegars. **Why?** Most vinegar is made from barley, which contains gluten. Balsamic vinegar is heralded as a low-fat dressing, but it contains sugar which doesn't equal a flat tummy.	**Better:** Organic lemon juice. **Why?** Lemon juice is packed with vitamin C and protects you from germs and bacteria.	**Best:** Organic apple cider vinegar. **Why?** It's full of natural bacteria-fighting enzymes, meaning it debloats you.
Bad: Processed cheese. **Why?** Most non-organic shop-bought cheeses are full of chemicals which can be stored in your fat tissue, making it hard for you to lose weight.	**Better:** Organic cheese. **Why?** Although it's still fatty, there are fewer toxins.	**Best:** Organic, locally produced goat's cheese. **Why?** This is easier to digest because it contains less lactose (which can cause bloating in some people).
Bad: Milk. **Why?** Most shop-bought, non-organic milk is filled with hormones.	**Better:** Organic milk. **Why?** Organic milk has no harsh synthetic chemicals added to it.	**Best:** Organic nut milks. **Why?** A great alternative to cow's milk as they don't contain lactose.
Bad: Regular yogurt. **Why?** Most shop-bought yogurts are full of sugar.	**Better:** Organic yogurt. **Why?** Organic yogurt is free from any harsh chemicals and preservatives.	**Best:** Organic full-fat yogurt. **Why?** The fat in this yogurt is great as it gives your body the feeling of fullness, plus it contains less sugar than 'low-fat' versions.
Bad: Aerosol whipped cream. **Why?** It's never organic, plus it's heavily processed and full of sugar.	**Better:** Regular cream. **Why?** It is natural, with no added chemicals to increase the shelf life.	**Best:** Organic cream. **Why?** Natural and pure.
Bad: Margarines. **Why?** They're usually full of chemicals and heavily processed (and dyed yellow to resemble butter).	**Better:** Olive spread. **Why?** Olives are a great source of essential fatty acids.	**Best:** Organic butter. **Why?** Natural and free of any preservatives or additives.
Bad: Ice cream. **Why?** Most shop-bought ice cream is full of sugar. It's a toxic, processed fat bomb heading for your stomach.	**Better:** Pure vanilla ice cream. **Why?** The fewer the ingredients, the better.	**Best:** Organic homemade frozen fruit purée. **Why?** Fruit is full of rich anti-oxidants and can be made in season.

CHAPTER 6

WORK OFF YOUR WOBBLY TUMMY

THIS CHAPTER WILL HELP YOU TO:

1. DISCOVER THE 10-MINUTE-A-DAY FAT BURNER
2. LEARN SIMPLE STOMACH-FLATTENING EXERCISES
3. FIND OUT WHY SIT-UPS WON'T FLATTEN YOUR TUMMY

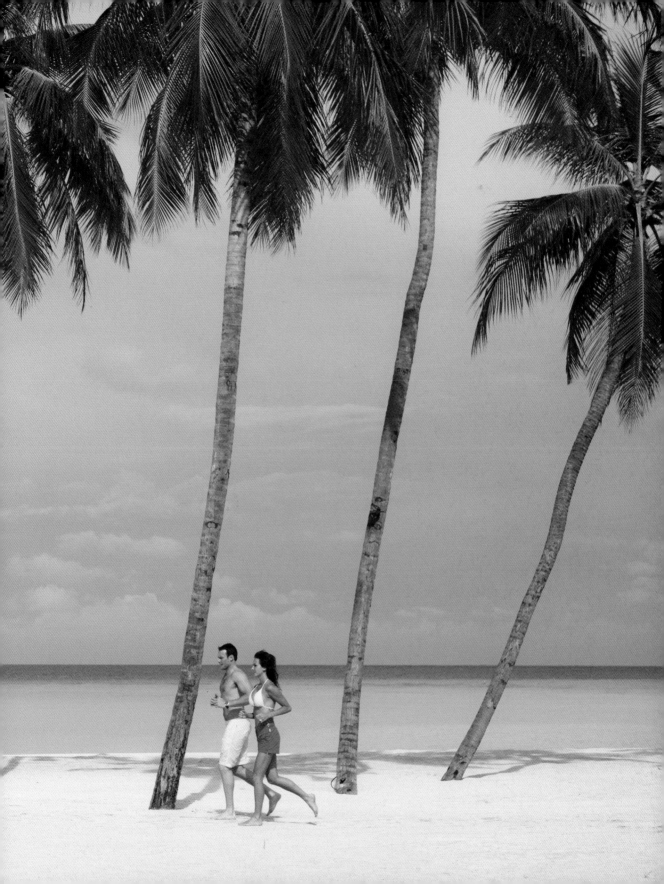

YOUR 14-DAY FLAT-STOMACH FITNESS PLAN

Monday, Wednesday and Friday:
* do the 10-minute fat burner
Tuesday and Thursday:
* do the fat-burning cardio (30 minutes)
Saturday and Sunday:
* rest.

During the 14-day flat-tummy eating plan (see Chapter 7), I want you to do the 10-minute fat burner plan detailed in this chapter. It involves 6 exercises (explained on pp. 69–73), each of which takes less than 2 minutes and involves a certain number of 'reps' (repetitions). Do the required number of reps, then move on to the next exercise. You need to do the 10-minute fat burner three times a week, with a day off in between. For ease, I'm going to say do it on a Monday, Wednesday and Friday. But you can change this according to fit in with your schedule, just as long as you keep a day between workouts. On the remaining two days (again, I'll say Tuesday and Thursday, but it's up to you when you do them), I want you do to 30 minutes of fat-burning cardio, which is explained on p. 71. Here goes . . .

*top tip
Commitment is the key to success – never give up no matter what, keep going!

THE 10-MINUTE FAT BURNER

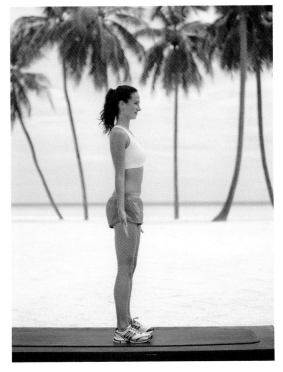
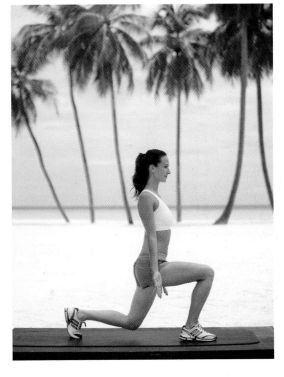

1. The forward lunge

Why? This is one of the best exercises for developing leg strength, plus it also works your stomach muscles. The legs constitute a huge muscle group, and the more you work them the more your muscles have to work and the more fat you burn. Plus, because you need to steady yourself, your abdominals get a great workout. The result? A very lean tummy.

✳ Stand with perfect posture with palms and both feet facing out, hip-width apart.

✳ Set the core.

✳ Step forward and lunge with one leg, as shown. Your front shin should be straight and perpendicular to the floor.

✳ Push up with the front leg and return to standing position.

✳ Repeat 12 times on each leg (24 reps in total).

*it's easy

Remember my 10-second rule to good posture: stand up straight, keep your back straight, with your ears over your shoulders and shoulders over your hips. Look straight ahead and think tall, right through your spine and through the top of your head. Not only will this intensify your workouts, it'll also make you look a dress size slimmer!

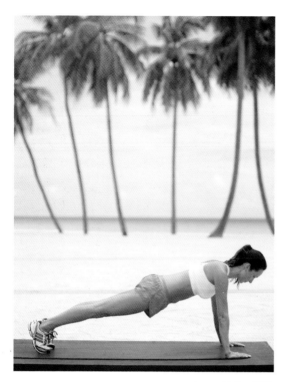
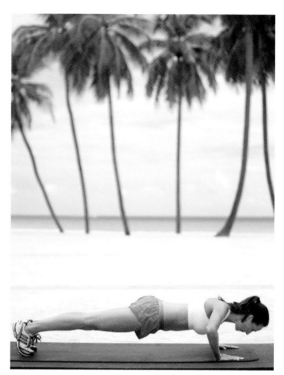

2. The perfect push-up

Why? This exercise is one of the best for working the core, making it a great tummy flattener. It also works your arms, legs and back.

* Set your hands one and a half shoulder widths apart and in line with your nipples, not with your shoulders. Keep your legs straight with the weight of your body distributed through your hands and toes.

* Keep your ears, shoulders and hips in alignment.

* Contract your stomach muscles.

* Lower yourself so your nose almost touches the ground, keeping your body straight, then lift back up to the starting position.

* Remember to keep your head up (if you drop your head, you'll have to work harder at 'carrying' it), and your belly button drawn in.

* Breathe out as you push up to start position, and in as you lower yourself down.

* Repeat 20 times.

*note

If you find this too difficult, start in the same position as above but with your arms on a chair or your sofa. The higher up your arms are, or the less horizontal the body is, the easier the push-up.

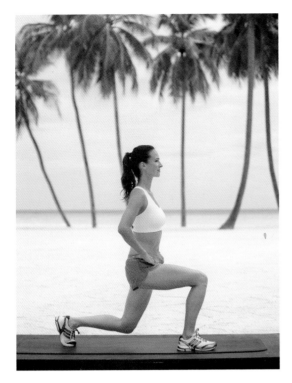

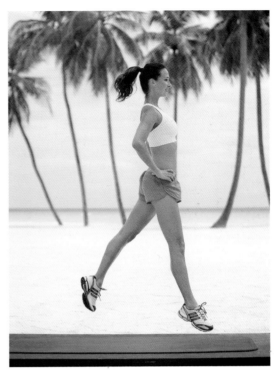

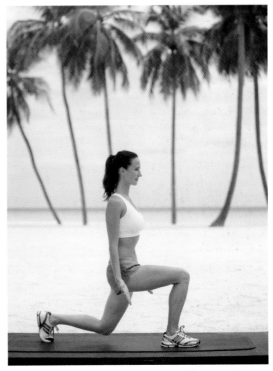

3. The lunge jump

Why? This exercise turns the forward lunge up a notch. The jump makes huge demands on the muscles, which burns more calories. The landing requires good stability and abdominal control.

✳ Start off in the lunge position (as shown) with your hands on your hips, then slowly lower yourself down and as you rise up, jump.

✳ Slowly and softly land back in the lunge position.

✳ Repeat 10 times on each leg (20 reps in total).

Fat-burning cardio
✳ 3 minutes: brisk walking
✳ 2 minutes: jogging (where you can still hold a conversation without getting out of breath).
✳ 1 minute: go sprinting (as fast as you can)
✳ Do this 8 times (so a total of 24 minutes).
✳ 5 minutes: brisk walking.

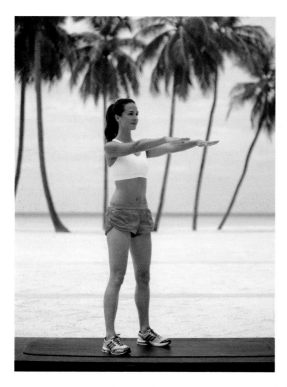

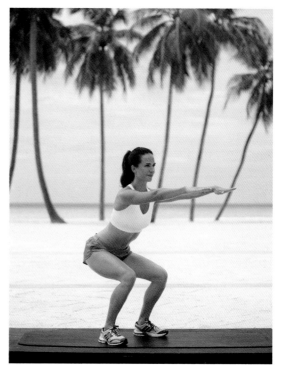

4. The squat

Why? This is an all-round great exercise and targets the butt and stomach muscles.

✳ Take a comfortable stance, keeping your feet shoulder-width apart, wider if necessary.

✳ Hold your arms out straight in front of you, parallel to the floor.

✳ Point your toes out slightly and make sure your knees stay aligned with your second toe; do not fall forwards or inwards when squatting. Keep your weight in your heels.

✳ Keeping your heels on the floor, lower yourself until your thighs are at least parallel with the floor. Stick your butt out.

✳ Go as low as you comfortably can while maintaining perfect posture (straight back, ears over shoulders).

✳ Push up through your heels and return to a standing position.

✳ Repeat 20 times.

5. The triceps dip with feet elevated (see p. 138 for pics)

Why? Along with the tummy and butt, the arms are another main concern for women. The normal bench/chair triceps dip requires you to have your feet on the floor. When you elevate your feet, it places more stress on the arms and also on your abdominals, making them work harder.

✳ Start by holding a bench with your feet slightly elevated. Set the core and then slowly lower yourself by bending from the elbows so they go backwards and remain close to your side.

✳ Once your forearms have touched your biceps, straighten your arms back to the start position.

✳ Ensure that you keep your chest up and you look straight ahead and not down.

✳ Repeat 20 times.

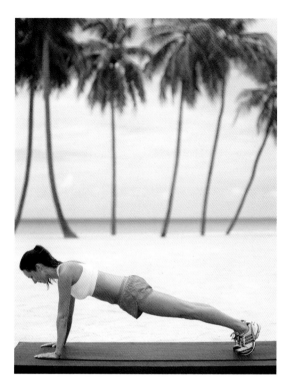

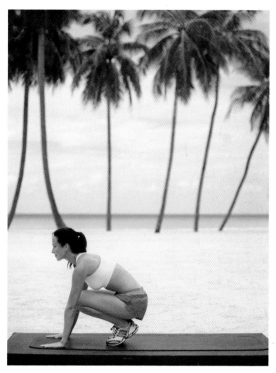

6. The burpie

Why? This is a great exercise as you need to use almost every muscle in your body and it burns lots of calories. The constant moving and jumping is a great abdominal workout which will tone all of your abdominal muscles.

✳ Start in a push-up position (see p. 70) with weight equally distributed between your hands and feet.

✳ Jump your feet towards your hands, then stand straight up with your hands in the air and jump. As you land, ensure that the weight of your body is equally distributed between your feet and that your landing is soft.

✳ Once you have finished the jump, place your hands on the floor beside your feet and then jump your feet back into the original start position, keeping your back straight when jumping back, and your abs tight.

✳ Repeat 20 times.

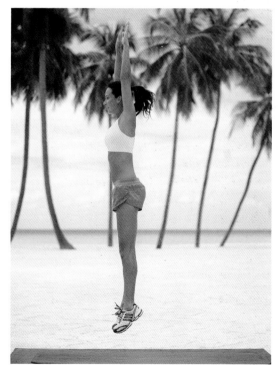

YOUR FLAT-STOMACH MAINTENANCE PROGRAMME

After the 14-day fitness plan, you can do the following programmes. Start at Level 1 (unless you're particularly fit and exercise regularly anyway), and after 4 weeks you should be aiming to work up to Level 2, then on to Level 3. It should take approximately 4 weeks to get to grips with each level, though it may take less (or more) time – just do whatever feels comfortable.

LEVEL 1

Monday, Wednesday and Friday:
* do the sequence of exercises below

Tuesday and Thursday:
* do the cardio exercises explained on p. 78

Exercise sequence
1) Squat curl press
2) Push-up with rotation (6 each side)
3) Standing W combo
4) Floor reverse crunches

How often? 12 reps per exercise with a 45-second rest after each. Complete 4 circuits.

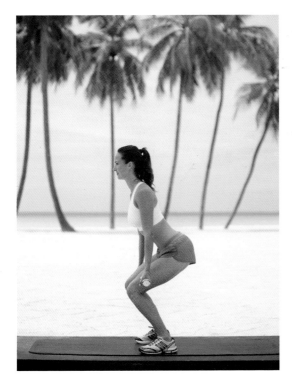

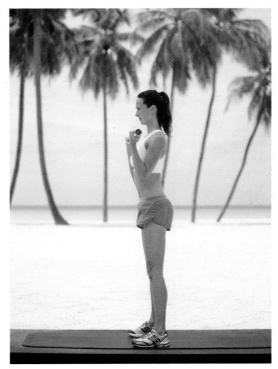

1. Squat curl press

✳ Take a comfortable stance, keeping your feet shoulder-width apart.

✳ Hold a pair of dumbbells in each hand with your palms facing out.

✳ Point your toes out slightly and make sure your knees stay aligned with your second toe; do not fall forwards or inwards when squatting. Keep your weight in your heels.

✳ Keeping your heels on the floor, lower yourself until your thighs are at least parallel with the floor. Stick your butt out. Go as low as you comfortably can, while maintaining perfect posture (straight back, ears over shoulders).

✳ Push up through your heels to return to standing.

✳ Once completed, slowly curl your arms so your palms are in line with your shoulders.

✳ With your hands level with your shoulders, turn your palms to face out and then press weights above your head in line with your ears.

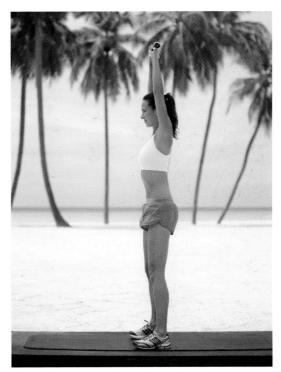

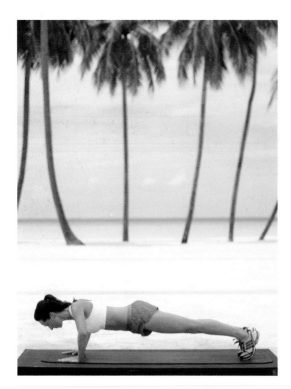

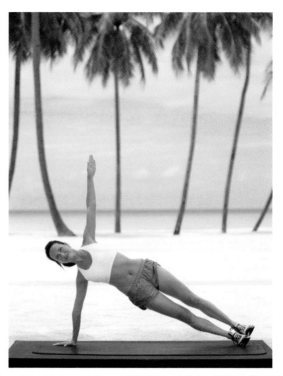

2. Push-up with rotation

＊ Get into the push-up position. Set your hands one and a half shoulder widths apart and in line with your nipples, not your shoulders. Keep your legs straight with your weight distributed through your hands and toes.

＊ Keep your ears, shoulders and hips in alignment.

＊ Contract your stomach muscles.

＊ Lower yourself so your nose almost touches the ground, keeping your body straight, then lift back up to start position.

＊ Once you reach the top position, rotate on your side, lifting your arm in to the air over your head so that all your body weight is on one arm and both feet.

＊ Hold for one second and then return to the start position.

＊ Keep your head up and your belly button drawn in.

＊ Breathe out as you push up to the start position, and in as you lower yourself down.

3. Standing W (opposite)

＊ Stand bent over at the waist with your back flat and chest up and feet shoulder-width apart.

＊ Draw your shoulder blades back and down and lift your elbows to the sky as they bend to 90 degrees, and rotate your hands to the sky in line with your ears.

＊ Raise your arms above your head, palms still facing forwards.

＊ Reverse the steps back to the start position.

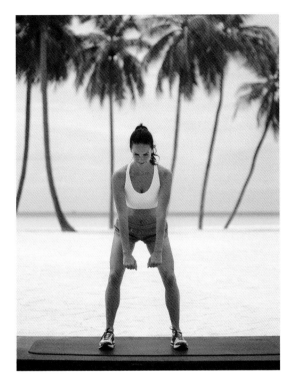
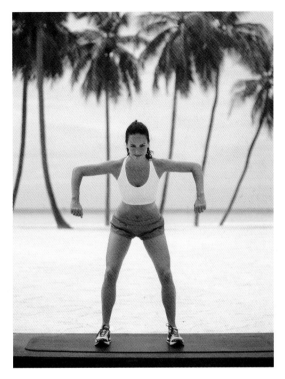
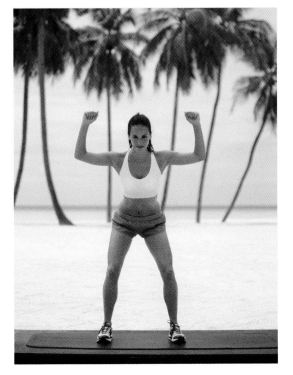
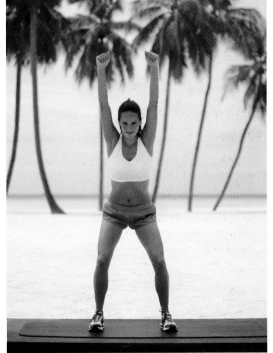

4. Floor reverse crunches

✳ Lie on your back with your legs straight up, your heels pointing towards the ceiling, arms outstretched at your sides and palms facing down.

✳ Slowly tighten your abs and rotate your pelvis slightly back and down.

✳ Lift your legs up towards the roof, so your lower back comes off the floor, then lower it slowly back down.

*reminder

When doing abdominal exercises, gently draw your belly into the spine. This will help to stabilise the spine and increase the work on the abs.

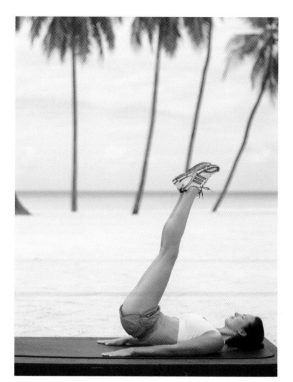

CARDIO LEVEL 1

✳ 3 minutes: brisk walking.
✳ 2 minutes: jogging (where you can still hold a conversation without getting out of breath).
✳ 1 minute: sprinting (go as fast as you can).
✳ Repeat the above 4–5 times.
✳ Have a 5-minute cool-down (walking and getting your breath back).

*top tip

Focus on the 'Big Bang' exercises. They shed extra pounds because they have such a high calorific demand. Big Bang exercises include lunges, chin-ups and triceps dips.

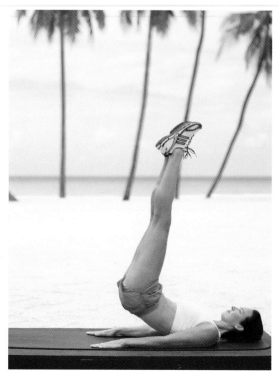

LEVEL 2

Monday, Wednesday and Friday:
* do the sequence of exercises below
Tuesday and Thursday:
* do the cardio exercises on p. 84.

Exercise sequence:
1) Static lunge-overhead triceps extensions (10 per leg)
2) Narrow-grip push-ups
3) Squat bent-over row
4) Side-bridge hold with hip drops (5 hip drops each side)
How often? 15 reps of each exercise. Have a 60-second rest after completing exercises 1–4. Do 5 circuits.

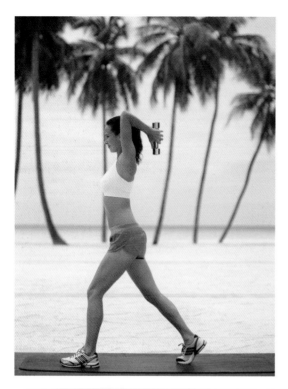

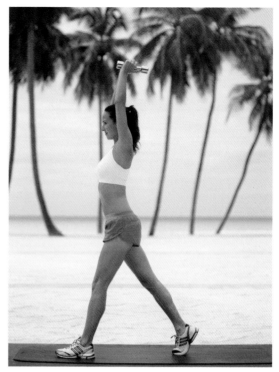

1. Static lunge-overhead triceps extensions

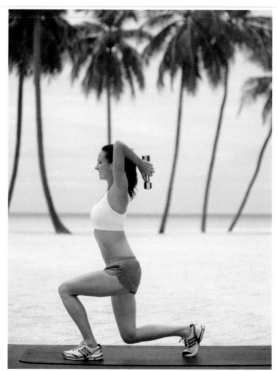

✳ Stand with perfect posture with your arms raised above your head holding dumbbells, palms facing.

✳ Both feet should face forwards, hip-width apart with straight front shins.

✳ Contract your stomach muscles.

✳ Lower your body by bending your back knee at the same time, bending your elbows with your hands going behind your head. Your back knee should just touch the floor.

✳ Push up, putting weight through the heel of the front foot at the same time straightening your arms.

3. Narrow-grip push-ups

✻ Get into the push-up position. Set your hands in line with your shoulders and in line with your nipples, not your shoulders and keep your legs straight with your weight distributed through hands and toes.

✻ Keep your ears, shoulders and hips in alignment.

✻ Contract your stomach muscles.

✻ Lower yourself so your nose almost touches the ground, keeping your body straight and elbows tucked into your sides, then lift back up to the start position.

✻ Hold for 1 second, then return to the start position.

✻ Remember to keep your head up and belly button drawn in.

✻ Breathe out as you push up to the start position, and in as you lower yourself down.

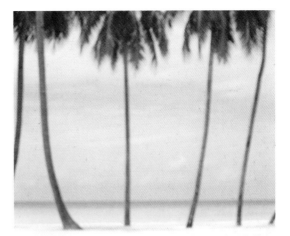
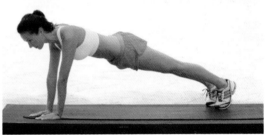
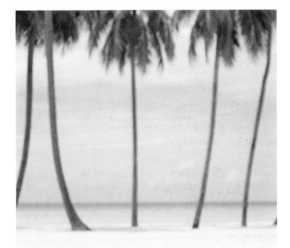
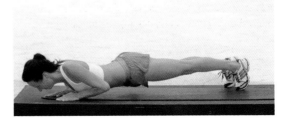

*top tip

Focus on the 'Big Bang' exercises. Make sure you focus your mind on your abdominal muscles.

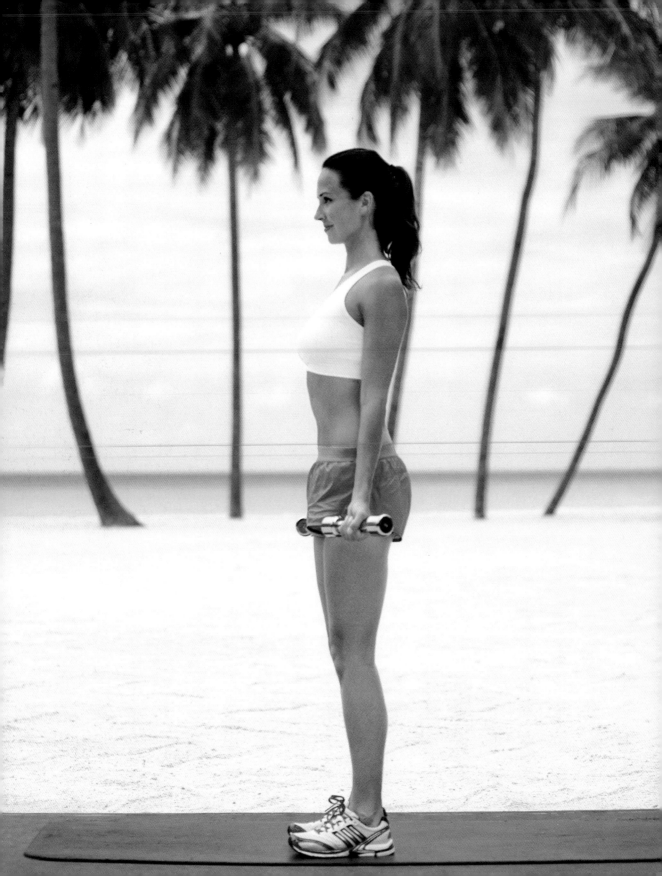

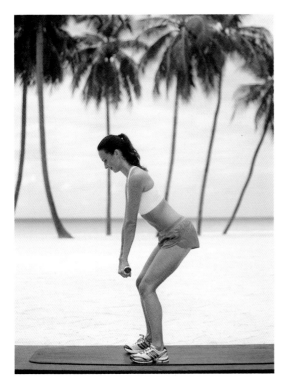 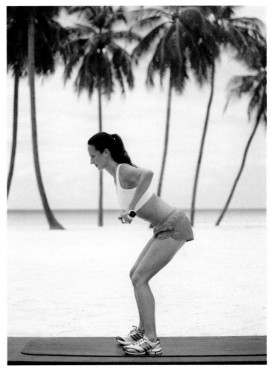

2. Squat bent-over row

✳ Take a comfortable stance, keeping your feet shoulder-width apart, wider if necessary. Hold the dumbbells in each hand with palms facing each other.

✳ Point your toes out slightly and make sure your knees stay aligned with your second toe; do not fall forwards or inwards when squatting. Keep your weight in your heels.

✳ Keeping your heels on the floor, lower yourself until your thighs are at least parallel with the floor. Stick your butt out. Go as low as you comfortably can with perfect posture (straight back, ears over shoulders).

✳ Keeping your knees slightly bent, move your hips slightly forwards (hinged over waist) keeping your back straight, chest up with arms out in front of the body.

✳ Slowly contract your abdominals and shoulder blades and row the dumbbells towards your chest, keeping your elbows close to your sides.

✳ Slowly lower, ensuring correct posture.

✳ Push up through your heels and return to standing.

*top tip
Using weights accelerates
the fat-burning process.

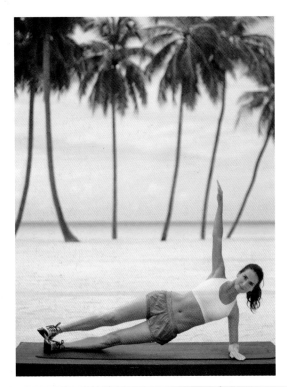
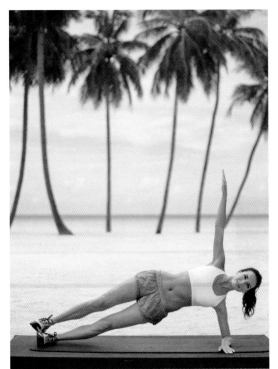

4. Side-bridge hold with hip drops

✳ Lie on your side with your forearm on the ground and your elbow under your shoulder and your other arm raised into the air.

✳ Push your forearm away from your body, keeping your elbow under your shoulder, lifting your hips into the air in a straight line and keeping your abs tight.

✳ Return to the start position in a controlled manner.

CARDIO LEVEL 2

✳ 3 minutes: brisk walking.
✳ 1½ minutes: jogging (where you can still hold a conversation without getting out of breath).
✳ 1 minute: sprinting (go as fast as you can).
✳ Repeat the above 5–6 times.
✳ Have a 5-minute cool-down (walking and getting your breath back).

*top tip

If your neck hurts while you're doing crunches, you may have an imbalance between your abdominal muscles and your neck. Just place your tongue behind your front teeth when crunching, with your mouth closed. This will help to stabilise your neck muscles so you can then train your abs even harder.

LEVEL 3

Monday, Wednesday and Friday:
* do the sequence of exercises below.
Tuesday and Thursday:
* do the cardio exercises on p. 88.

Exercise sequence:
1. Arms-raised forward lunges (15 per leg)
2. Push-up burpies
3. Hammer curls – upright row
4. Feet-elevated crunches

How often? 20 reps per exercise with a 60-second rest
after exercises 1–4 are complete. Do 6 circuits.

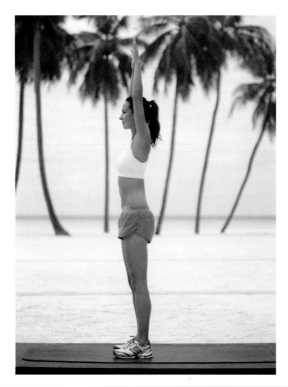

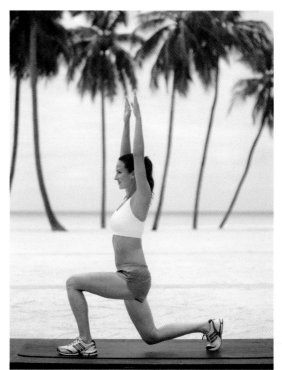

1. Arms-raised forward lunges

✳ Stand with perfect posture, hands above your head, palms facing forwards.

✳ Both feet should face out straight and be hip-width apart.

✳ Set the core.

✳ Step forwards into the lunge with your arms staying straight above your head. Your front shin should be straight and perpendicular to the floor.

✳ Push up back to the start position with your front leg returning to a standing position and then step forward with the opposite leg.

2. Push-up burpies

✳ Start in a push-up position with your body weight equally distributed between your hands and feet. Perform a standard push-up and once completed . . .

✳ . . . jump your feet towards, then stand straight up with your hands in the air and jump – as you land, ensure that the weight is equally distributed between your feet and that your landing is soft.

✳ Once you have finished the jump, place your hands on the floor beside your feet and then jump your feet back into the original start position. Keep your back straight when jumping back and your abs tight.

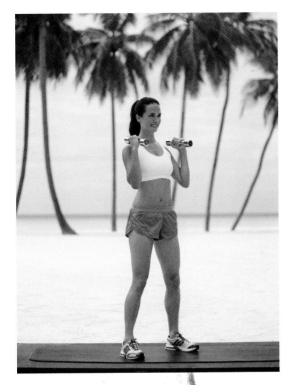

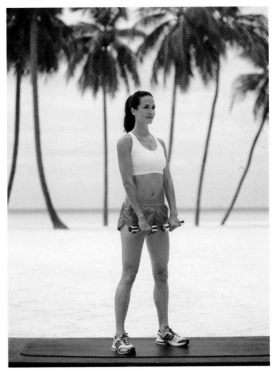

3. Hammer curls – upright row

✳ Take a comfortable stance, keeping your feet shoulder-width apart, wider if necessary.

✳ Hold your dumbbells in each hand, palms facing each other.

✳ Slowly curl your arms so your palms are in line with your shoulders, then return to the start position.

✳ Now turn your hands so your palms are facing your thighs.

✳ Pull the dumbbells to the front of your shoulders with your elbows leading out to the sides.

✳ Allow your wrists to flex, as the dumbbells rise upwards. Then return to the start position.

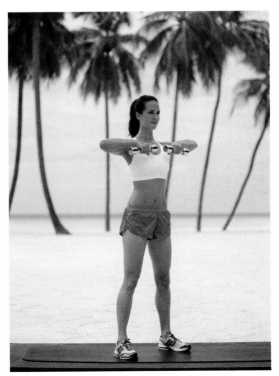

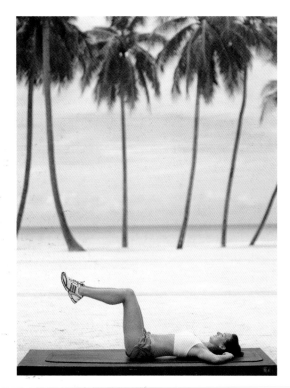

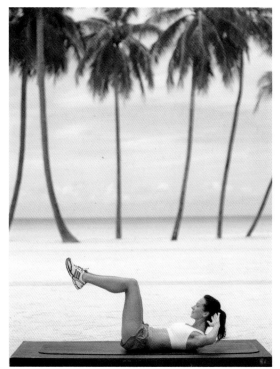

4. Feet-elevated crunches

✳ Lie on your back with knees bent at 90 degrees, heels off the floor and toes pointing towards the ceiling.

✳ Place your fingers behind your ears with your elbows out and contract your abs. Lift your shoulder blades off the floor.

✳ At the same time, press your heels towards the ceiling, creating a 'U' shape with your torso.

✳ Return to the start position.

CARDIO LEVEL 3

✳ 3 minutes: brisk walking.
✳ 1½ minutes: jogging (where you can still hold a conversation without getting out of breath).
✳ 1 minute: sprinting (go as fast as you can).
✳ Repeat the above 6–7 times.
✳ Have a 5-minute cool-down (walking and getting your breath back).

*top tip
Bored of running. Get on your bike or kick a boxing bag.

*top tip

Work your pelvic-floor muscles. They're your body's natural corset (along with your abdominals), so if you work these regularly, you'll get a taut lower stomach. Your pelvic-floor muscles are the ones you would use if you were trying to stop the flow of urine. Squeeze and clench them (as if you're stopping the flow) up to 15 times. You may need to work up to this number. Do 15–20 squeezes, 5 times a day. You can do them anywhere and nobody will suspect. Pregnancy weakens your pelvic-floor muscles, so it's really important to do them after you've had children.

BAD, BETTER, BEST GUIDE TO EXERCISE

BAD	BETTER	BEST
Bad: Only doing aerobic classes, such as step or spin, for weight loss. **Why?** Pure cardio increases cortisol levels and can make you fatter.	**Better:** Mixing cardio with classes such as Body Bump or weights. **Why?** These have a resistance element which puts demand on the muscles and helps to build lean muscle mass.	**Best:** Free weights and interval training (this is where you do short bursts of cardio, mixed with slower ones – running fast, then jogging, then running fast, for example. **Why?** Interval training requires short bursts of energy, which burns serious amounts of calories and doesn't increase your cortisol levels.
Bad: Running on the treadmill. **Why?** This is lazy as the treadmill pulls the back leg.	**Better**: Running outside. **Why?** The bumpy surface you get outside requires your feet and ankles to stabilise the body, and your abs have to work to keep you upright.	**Best:** Running on sand. **Why?** The sand is perfect as it really works your legs – you burn so many more calories – and even better barefoot. OK, so you may not get the chance to run on sand that often, but when you do, give it a try.
Bad: Static stretching before exercise. **Why?** This can cause more damage to a muscle.	**Better:** Doing a dynamic warm-up before exercise. **Why?** Dynamic movements mimic the movements of the sports.	**Best**: Foam rolling release and dynamic warm-up. **Why?** Foam rolling is a great way to start an exercise programme as it helps to loosen the tissue around the muscles (see www.bodyism.com).
Bad: Not eating before exercise. **Why?** Your body needs fuel to exercise, just like a car needs petrol to drive.	**Better:** Eating 60 minutes before training. **Why?** This will allow your body time to digest.	**Best:** Having a Bodyism Body Brilliance pre-workout drink (visit www.bodyism.com) or a light snack of berries and a couple of nuts 30 minutes before you begin to exercise. **Why?** Perfect nutrient ratio for optimum energy and fat burning.
Bad: Having a sports drink before exercise. **Why?** They're too full of sugar and additives.	**Better:** Water mixed with a little fruit juice. **Why?** A natural, chemical-free drink.	**Best:** Water with a pinch of salt. **Why?** The salt helps bring the water into your cells as you exercise.

BAD	BETTER	BEST
Bad: Drinking a caffeine energy drink before exercise. **Why?** They are full of artificial chemicals.	**Better:** Drinking vitamin drinks with natural caffeine such as guarana or Yerba Mate. **Why?** A better source of caffeine.	**Best:** 30 minutes before exercise have an organic black espresso with a sprinkle of cinnamon. **Why?** Perfect amount of caffeine with the fat-burning benefits of cinnamon.
Bad: Isolation training for weight loss – for example repeated biceps curls. **Why?** Inefficient fat-burning and can lead to a bulky physique.	**Better:** Standing or kneeling biceps curls. **Why?** Free weight isolation exercise is better as it requires more stability, which works your abs harder.	**Best:** Chin-ups. **Why?** Exercises like these work several muscle groups, not just one.
Bad: Knee extensions on a gym machine. **Why?** This only works one set of muscles	**Better:** Squats using your body weight. **Why?** A big exercise improves joint stability and burns buckets of fat.	**Best:** Dumbbell squats. **Why?** By holding weights, you're increasing demand on your muscles and burning more fat.

WHY SIT-UPS ALONE ARE NOT ENOUGH

Sit-ups alone won't take inches off your waist or flatten your stomach. When you do hundreds of crunches your abdominal muscles (especially the rectus abdominus – the 'six pack' muscles) tends to overdevelop and you can get a distension of the tummy. I've seen this hundreds of times with my clients.

Plus, if you're doing lots of sit-ups with the wrong technique (again, something I've seen hundreds of times) this will place excessive strain on your hip flexors (the group of muscles around your hips). This can cause a Donald Duck-style posture – the kind that gives you a sticking-out bottom, a curved back and a little 'pouch belly'. Not the look you're after, I'm sure!

The best way to exercise your way to a flat stomach is to combine sit-ups (done properly) with other types of exercises that all work together to tighten, strengthen and flatten your stomach. Sit-ups alone won't do a thing!

*top tip

Flexible hip flexors make for a flatter tummy and prevent back pain, so make sure you stretch them. Kneel down on both knees with your back straight. Step forward with one leg, putting your hands on the thigh out in front of you. Slide your back leg as far back as you can until you feel a stretch in your hips. Maintaining this posture, shift your body slightly forward. Exhale and hold for 3 seconds. Repeat 5 times on each leg.

CHAPTER 7

THE 14-DAY FLAT TUMMY FAST! EATING PLAN AND RECIPES

RECIPES BY CLARA GRACE PAUL

THIS CHAPTER WILL HELP YOU TO:

1. DEVELOP GOOD EATING HABITS FOR LIFE
2. LEARN HOW TO STAVE OFF HUNGER
3. DE-BLOAT IN DAYS

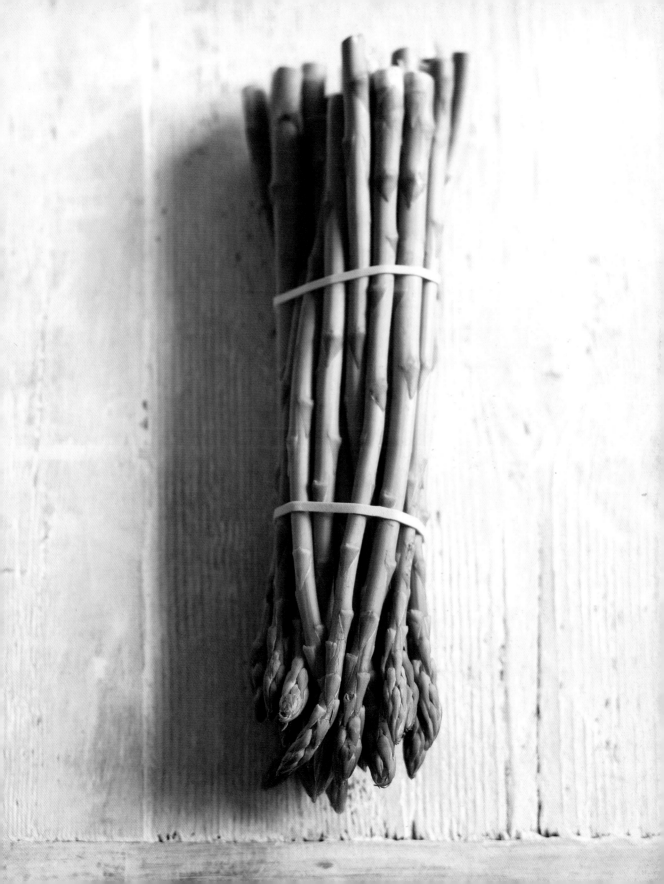

THE 14-DAY EATING PLAN

When you feel ready to start, follow this 14-day plan. It's best to start on a weekend, when you have more time on your hands to get everything ready. Plus you won't feel so stressed or rushed, which will mean you'll be less likely to supplement the plan with a quick coffee or a mid-afternoon chocolate bar.

You can swap meals around (have Day 1 breakfast on Day 2, for example), but try to stick to the plan as much as possible. You shouldn't feel hungry, but if you do, just increase your green vegetable portions and make sure you're drinking enough water (at least 2–3 litres of still, filtered water a day).

Where possible (and if you can afford it), go for organic ingredients – especially when it comes to eggs (free-range are also good) and meat.

DAY 1

Breakfast: a 3-egg-white omelette filled with ¼ cup mixed peppers and a handful of spinach.

Snack, mid-morning: 100g chicken with ½ red pepper, sliced.

Lunch: 1 grilled chicken breast, a salad with mixed leaves, red peppers and green beans, drizzled with ¼ tablespoon olive oil.

Snack, mid-afternoon: 100g turkey breast with ¼ cucumber.

Dinner: 100g grilled chicken breast with steamed broccoli (unlimited amount).

DAY 2

Breakfast: 1 baked chicken breast with a handful of kale – either steam or lightly stir-fry it.

Snack, mid-morning: 100g turkey breast and ½ green pepper, sliced.

Lunch: 1 haddock fillet (either grill or bake it) with a mixed green salad, drizzled with ½ tablespoon walnut oil.

Snack, mid-afternoon: 100g turkey breast with 75g raw or lightly steamed broccoli.

Dinner: 1 salmon steak topped with chopped dill, served with a large portion of steamed green beans.

COOKING METHODS

You can choose your own cooking methods, but remember that you'll see quicker results if you steam or bake the vegetables and grill or bake the meat/fish. With vegetables, the less time you spend cooking them, the more nutrients will remain. Overcooked vegetables don't contain as many nutrients as lightly steamed ones.

DAY 3	DAY 4	DAY 5	DAY 6
Breakfast: 4–6 scallops (pan-fry them quickly, 2 minutes each side) or another white fish with a portion of steamed asparagus.	**Breakfast:** 3 scrambled eggs (1 whole egg and 2 egg whites) with grilled tomatoes, mixed with 1 portion of green beans.	**Breakfast:** 200g turkey breast with ¼ avocado and ¼ cucumber, sliced.	**Breakfast:** 1 grilled haddock fillet with a portion of roasted peppers and courgettes.
Snack, mid-morning: 100g chicken breast with ½ yellow pepper, sliced.	**Snack, mid-morning:** 100g turkey slices with ¼ cucumber, sliced.	**Snack, mid-morning:** 2 hard-boiled eggs with ½ red pepper, sliced.	**Snack, mid-morning:** 100g chicken with 1 tomato, sliced.
Lunch: 1 grilled chicken breast with garden salad, drizzled with ½ tablespoon macadamia nut oil.	**Lunch:** baked cod fillet (roughly 150g) with salad, including tomato and baby spinach, and ½ tablespoon flaxseed oil.	**Lunch:** 150g grilled prawns with a green salad and tomatoes, drizzled with ½ tablespoon pumpkin seed oil.	**Lunch:** 150g turkey with a green salad and steamed broccoli, drizzled with ½ tablespoon olive oil.
Snack, mid-afternoon: 100g turkey slices with ¼ avocado.	**Snack, mid-afternoon:** 100g chicken breast with ½ grilled courgette.	**Snack, mid-afternoon:** 100g turkey breast with 5 almonds.	**Snack, mid-afternoon:** 100g chicken with 5 pecan nuts.
Dinner: 2 lamb cutlets or 1 lamb steak (grilled) with a large portion of steamed broccoli and spinach.	**Dinner:** 100g chicken breast stir-fry made with ½ teaspoon coconut oil and green vegetables.	**Dinner:** 100g chicken breast with a portion of steamed broccoli.	**Dinner:** 150–200g steak with a portion of steamed green beans and broccoli.

WHAT IS A 100G

If you don't have scales to weigh your portions, here's a rough guide to the measurements given in the 14-day plan:

100g chicken = two-thirds the size of a regular breast or the palm of your hand (minus fingers).

100g smoked salmon = the size of your outstretched hand (including fingers)

100g beef fillet = the size of a tennis ball.

DAY 7

Breakfast: 3-egg-white omelette filled with grilled tomatoes and served with a portion of steamed spinach.

Snack, mid-morning: 100g turkey with 5 Brazil nuts.

Lunch: 150g chicken breast with steamed asparagus and a green salad.

Snack, mid-afternoon: 100g turkey with ¼ cucumber, sliced.

Dinner: a stir-fry made with 100g prawns, 5 scallops and mixed vegetables, cooked with ½ teaspoon of coconut oil.

DAY 8

Breakfast: 100g chicken breast with ½ yellow pepper and ¼ avocado.

Snack, mid-morning: 100g turkey and 4 macadamia nuts.

Lunch: 3-egg-white omelette filled with ¼ cup mixed peppers, and served with a portion of spinach.

Snack, mid-afternoon: 100g turkey with a portion of steamed green beans.

Dinner: 1 cod fillet baked with a green salad and tomatoes, drizzled with ½ tablespoon pumpkin seed oil.

DAY 9

Breakfast: 100g smoked salmon and a portion of spinach.

Snack, mid-morning: 100g chicken breast and 6 pecan nuts.

Lunch: 1 chicken breast with a portion of roasted peppers and courgettes.

Snack, mid-afternoon: 2 hard-boiled eggs and ½ cucumber, sliced.

Dinner: a grilled duck breast (skin removed) served with steamed Chinese broccoli.

DAY 10

Breakfast: 150g turkey breast, ½ green pepper and ¼ avocado.

Snack, mid-morning: 100g chicken breast and 12 cashew nuts.

Lunch: baked sea bass with a mixed green salad.

Snack, mid-afternoon: 100g chicken breast and ½ sliced tomato.

Dinner: 100–200g fillet steak with steamed broccoli.

DAY 11	DAY 12	DAY 13	DAY 14
Breakfast: 3 scrambled egg whites served with grilled asparagus.	**Breakfast:** 1 baked chicken breast with a portion of spinach.	**Breakfast:** 4–6 scallops with a portion of steamed broccoli.	**Breakfast:** 3 scrambled eggs (one yolk, two whites) mixed with a portion of steamed spinach and a sliced grilled tomato.
Snack, mid-morning: 100g turkey breast and ¼ avocado.	**Snack, mid-morning:** 100g turkey and 5 walnuts.	**Snack, mid-morning:** 100g sliced turkey breast with ½ red pepper, sliced.	**Snack, mid morning:** 100g chicken slices with 5 hazelnuts.
Lunch: 150g grilled prawns served with a green salad and tomatoes, drizzled with ½ tablespoon flaxseed oil.	**Lunch:** 150g turkey breast with a green salad and a portion of steamed mangetout, drizzled with ½ tablespoon olive oil.	**Lunch:** 150g chicken with a bowl of garden salad and ¼ cucumber, sliced, and drizzled with ½ teaspoon of macadamia nut oil.	**Lunch:** 150g baked cod with a salad, including tomato and baby spinach drizzled with ½ tablespoon flaxseed oil.
Snack, mid-afternoon: 100g chicken breast with ½ yellow pepper.	**Snack, mid-afternoon:** 100g turkey breast and ¼ cucumber, sliced.	**Snack, mid-afternoon:** 100g sliced turkey breast with ¼ avocado.	**Snack, mid-afternoon:** 100g turkey slices with ½ green pepper, sliced.
Dinner: 1 grilled haddock fillet with roasted peppers, courgettes and kale.	**Dinner:** 1 salmon steak, topped with chopped dill, served with a portion of steamed Brussels sprouts and rocket salad.	**Dinner:** 1 lemon sole fillet with a portion of steamed green beans.	**Dinner:** 100–200g fillet steak with a portion of grilled asparagus and a portion of steamed spinach.

*top tip
Stick this plan on
your fridge as a
constant reminder,
then you won't be
tempted to stray.

FLAT-TUMMY FOODS YOU SHOULD KEEP IN YOUR KITCHEN

Meat
* Chicken
* Turkey
* Lamb
* Beef
* Duck

Vegetables
* Broccoli
* Spinach
* Asparagus
* Green beans
* Mangetout
* Kale
* Rocket
* Watercress
* Brussels sprouts
* Cucumber
* Courgettes
* Avocados
* Sweet Potatoes
* Leeks
* Peas
* Mushrooms

Herbs and flavours
* Garlic
* Ginger
* Fresh lemon
* Fresh lime
* Red clover
* Camomile
* Tarragon
* Dill
* Rosemary
* Sage
* Passion flower
* Cinnamon (this is great for lowering blood-sugar levels, which in turn reduces sugar cravings)

Fruit
* Blueberries
* Raspberries
* Blackberries
* Acai berries
* Melons

Dairy
(organic where you can afford it)
* Yogurt
* Eggs

Nuts, seeds and fats
* Almonds
* Pecans
* Walnuts
* Brazil nuts
* Pistachios
* Macadamias
* Chestnuts
* Sesame seeds
* Sunflower seeds
* Pumpkin seeds
* Linseeds (ground only)
* Coconut oil
* Olive oil (virgin cold-pressed – preferably not to cook with, but to drizzle over stuff, like salads, vegetables and meat/fish)
* Walnut oil
* Sesame oil
* Basil-infused olive oil
* Garlic-infused olive oil

COOKING THE CLEAN & LEAN WAY TO A FLATTER TUMMY

THE CLEANEST WAYS TO COOK:

Steaming

Steaming is one of the healthiest ways to cook fish, meat and vegetables as it retains nearly all the nutrients (and flavour) found in food and doesn't add any fat. As the name of the method suggests, the food doesn't come into contact with the water – just the steam that the water lets off. The most common way to do this is to suspend the food over boiling water with a steamer (this usually has holes in it to allow the steam through).

Blanching

This is a way of cooking vegetables that keeps them crisp and tender, while retaining lots of the nutrients. You boil them for a short amount of time, so that they're barely cooked, then you remove them from the heat, drain, then add them to a bowl of icy water. Wait until they're no longer warm, then quickly reheat them (either by boiling/steaming/ grilling for 30–60 seconds).

Grilling

This is a great way to cook meat and fish as the fat drips away from the food resting on a grill rack making it much healthier than frying or roasting.

Baking/roasting

There isn't any real difference between these two. They're methods of cooking meat, fish or vegetables using dry heat (your oven) which browns the food's exterior and cooks the middle.

AND THE WORST WAYS TO COOK:

Frying

Usually, this involves cooking foods with oil in a hot pan. Firstly, the oil soaks into the food, and secondly, because that fat is heated up it becomes less healthy (cold olive oil is far healthier than hot olive oil, for example).

Boiling

When you boil vegetables in water they lose many of their health-boosting nutrients. Blanching (see opposite) is OK because you're only boiling them for a short amount of time. But when you just boil your vegetables – for a long time – too many nutrients are lost.

Microwaving

This method may save you time during a hectic day and it's tempting when you're tired to zap something quickly, but it is not a method of cooking that I recommend. Some studies have found that it can destroy up to 97 per cent of the health-boosting antioxidants found in vegetables.

*reminder

The less you cook it, the more alive your food will be.

BREAKFASTS & SMOOTHIES

Serenity Shake

Ingredients
10g BodySerenity (www.bodyism.com)
250ml rice milk
1 teaspoon fresh camomile

Method
1. Mix all the ingredients together in a blender. Serve in a tall glass and drink immediately.

Cantaloupe with Seeded Yogurt

Ingredients
1 tablespoon toasted flaked almonds
1 tablespoon walnuts
1 tablespoon pumpkin seeds
200ml natural organic yogurt
1 cantaloupe melon, peeled, deseeded and cut into slices

Method
1. Mix the nuts and seeds into the yogurt and spoon over the melon slices.

Brilliance Shake

Ingredients
10g BodyBrilliance powder (www.bodyism.com)
250ml oat milk
1 banana or a handful of blueberries

Method
1. Mix all the ingredients together in a blender. Serve in a tall glass and drink immediately.

*top tip
This is a great treat to have every now and again, as cantaloupe is a great antioxidant.

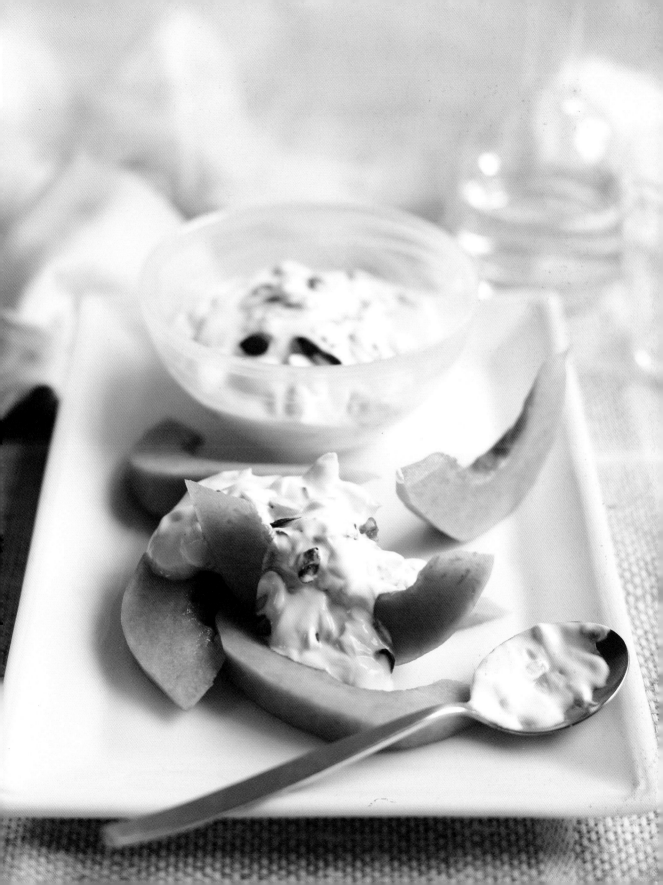

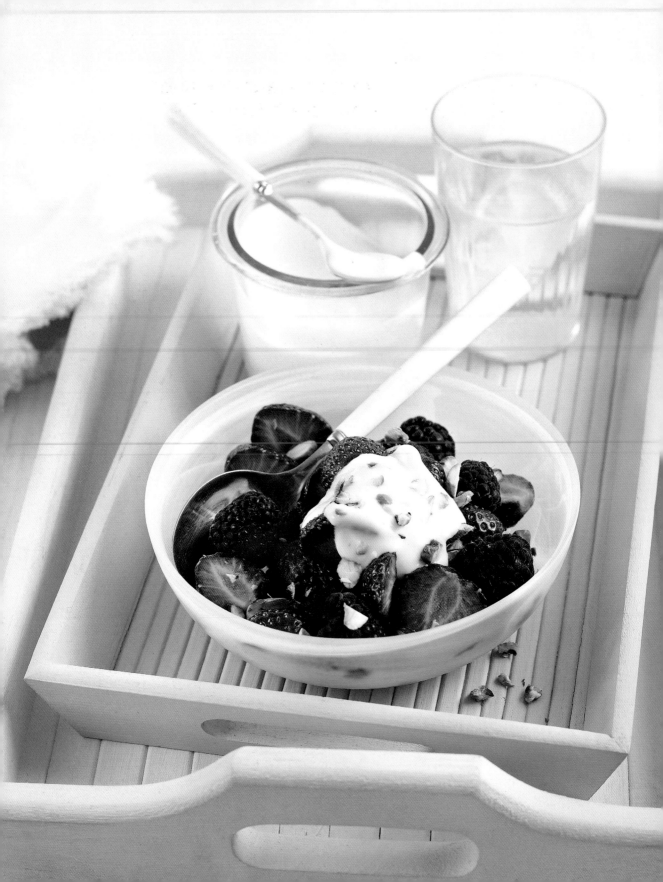

Red Berry Salad with Natural Yogurt

Serves 1

Ingredients

a large handful of both strawberries
  and raspberries
1 tablespoon pistachio nuts
1 tablespoon passion flower
2 tablespoons organic natural yogurt

Method

1. Mix the berries, pistachios, and passion flower together. Serve with yogurt.

Spinach and Tomato Omelette

Ingredients

1 tablespoon olive oil
2 large vine tomatoes, deseeded
  and chopped
1 bag of baby spinach
8 free-range organic eggs, beaten with
  salt and pepper

Method

1. Heat the oil in a large non-stick frying pan. Gently fry the tomatoes over a medium heat for about 4 minutes.

2. Add the spinach and cook until it starts to wilt.

3. Pour in the beaten eggs, pushing the edges into the middle and tilting the pan to distribute evenly.

4. After about 4 minutes, fold one half over and continue to cook for a further 3–4 minutes.

*see bodyism.com

Smoked Haddock and Watercress Omelette

Ingredients

8 free-range, organic eggs
2 naturally smoked haddock fillets,
  flaked or cut into chunks
1 bunch of watercress, chopped
salt and pepper

Method

1. Beat the eggs in a large bowl, then add all the other ingredients. Cook as for Spinach and Tomato Omelette.

The Super-skinny Smoothie

Serves 1

Ingredients

2 Brazil nuts
2 almonds
a handful of blueberries and raspberries
a scoop of Body Brilliance*
a scoop of Body Fibre Ultimate Clean*
1 glass of water/milk/rice milk/almond milk

Method

1. Mix all the ingredients together in a blender. Serve in a tall glass and drink immediately.

Super-skinny Fat-burning Drink

Ingredients:

Take 3 heaped tablespoons of cinnamon, ½ teaspoon of baking soda, and mix it with 900ml boiling water (or organic milk, or alternative milks, such as rice and almond). Strain it out and then put it in a jar with a lid on it. Once it's cooled down, put it in the fridge.
Drink 125–225ml a day. It helps with blood-sugar levels (so combats sugar cravings).

LUNCH & DINNER

Note: all recipes serve 4,
unless otherwise stated.

Chicken on a bed of Roasted Vegetables and Rocket

Ingredients
2 red onions
2 red peppers
2 yellow peppers
2 courgettes
2 tablespoons olive oil, plus extra
  for drizzling
1 tablespoon balsamic vinegar
4 skinless chicken breasts
2 garlic cloves, crushed
2 tablespoons sesame oil
1 tablespoon tamari soy sauce
1 large bag of rocket
1 bunch of basil

Method
1. Preheat the oven to 200°C/400°F/gas 6.

2. Cut all the vegetables into even slices/chunks and mix with the olive oil and balsamic vinegar. Place on a baking tray and bake for about 40 minutes.

3. Remove from the oven and rub the chicken breasts with the crushed garlic, sesame oil and tamari soy sauce. Bake for 25 minutes.

4. Cool slightly and slice on the diagonal.

5. Arrange the rocket on a flat platter. Scatter the roasted vegetables over the rocket, top with the sliced chicken. Pour over any cooking juices, drizzle with extra-virgin olive oil and scatter over whole basil leaves.

Sesame Seed and Fenugreek Chicken Wings

Ingredients
4 tablespoons sesame seeds
2 tablespoons sesame oil
1 tablespoon ground fenugreek
2 tablespoons organic maple syrup
3 garlic cloves, crushed
12 free-range chicken wings

Method
1. Mix together all the ingredients except the chicken in a large bowl. Marinate the chicken wings in the mixture overnigh or for at least 15 minutes.

2. Preheat the oven to 200°C/400°F/gas 6.

3. Bake the chicken wings in a roasting pan for approximately 30 minutes.

Always use organic meat as it is less likely to be packed with hormones that make your tummy fat.

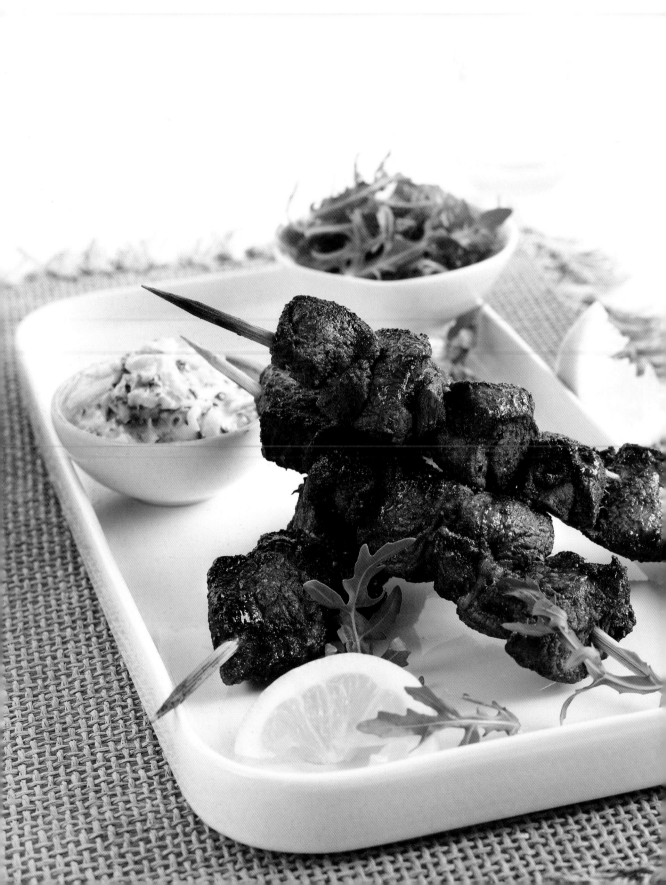

Greek Lamb Skewers with Courgette Tzatziki

Ingredients

600g lamb leg steaks, trimmed and cut
  into large chunks
2 tablespoons olive oil
1 teaspoon cinnamon
1 teaspoon ground coriander
½ cucumber
2 courgettes
1 small bunch of mint, finely chopped
300ml organic natural yogurt
zest of 1 lemon
juice of ½ lemon
rocket leaves, to serve
salt and pepper

Method

1. Rub the lamb with the olive oil, salt, pepper, cinnamon and coriander. Thread on to wooden skewers that have been soaked in water for 30 minutes.

2. Heat a grill/griddle pan to a medium heat.

3. Grate the cucumber and courgettes and mix in a bowl with the finely chopped mint leaves. Stir in the yogurt and lemon zest.

4. Grill the lamb for about 4 minutes on each side until cooked through and golden. Squeeze the lemon juice over the lamb and serve with the tzatziki and some peppery rocket.

Green Bean, Mangetout, Spinach and Macadamia Nut Salad

Ingredients

250g trimmed green beans
250g mangetout
1 large bag of baby spinach
1 tablespoon camomile
150g macadamia nuts, roughly chopped
2 tablespoons walnut oil
zest and juice of ½ lemon

Method

1. Blanch the green beans and mangetout in lightly salted boiling water for about 4 minutes, or until tender but with a bite. Drain and rinse under cold water.

2. Arrange the baby spinach on a serving platter. Layer the beans and mangetout on top and scatter over the camomile.

3. Sprinkle the chopped macadamia nuts over the top. Pour over the walnut oil and lemon juice and zest and serve immediately.

Mackerel is packed with omega 3 fatty acids which are great for your waistline.

Grilled Monkfish with Rosemary, Green Beans and Sprouting Broccoli

Ingredients

4 monkfish fillets, cut into chunks
2 tablespoons rosemary, finely chopped
1 tablespoon olive oil
200g green beans
200g purple sprouting broccoli
juice of 1 lemon
1 tablespoon walnut oil
salt and pepper

Method

1. Preheat the grill to medium.

2. Toss the monkfish in the rosemary, olive oil, salt and pepper. Then thread on to wooden skewers that have been soaked in water for 30 minutes.

3. Meanwhile, blanch the green beans and purple sprouting broccoli in salted water for about 4 minutes. Then drain and toss in the lemon juice and walnut oil. Season to taste.

4. Cook the monkfish under the hot grill for 5 minutes, turning regularly. Check that it is cooked through then serve with the vegetables, topped with lemon wedges.

Pan-fried Mackerel with Melon Salsa

Ingredients

4 regular-sized mackerel fillets
1 teaspoon ground cinnamon
1 teaspoon ground cumin
1 teaspoon ground coriander
4 vine tomatoes
1 red onion
1 red chilli
1 bunch of coriander
1 cantaloupe melon
juice of 1 lime
1 tablespoon coconut oil
½ teaspoon olive oil

Method

1. Lightly score the skin of the mackerel fillets. Mix the spices together and rub all over the mackerel fillets.

2. Dice the tomatoes and red onion, thinly slice the chilli, finely chop the coriander and peel, deseed and dice the melon. Mix all of these together in a bowl.

3. Whisk the lime juice and the coconut oil and pour over the salsa. Mix well. Set aside until needed.

4. Heat a non-stick frying pan over a medium heat. Pour in the olive oil. Lay the mackerel fillets in the pan, skin-side down, and cook for 5 minutes. Flip over and cook for a further 5 minutes. Serve with the salsa.

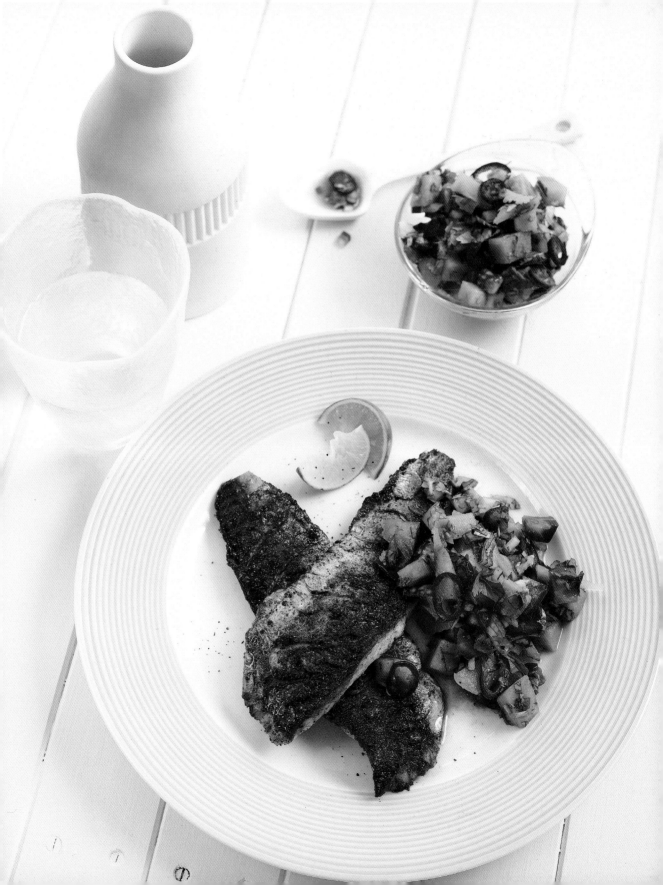

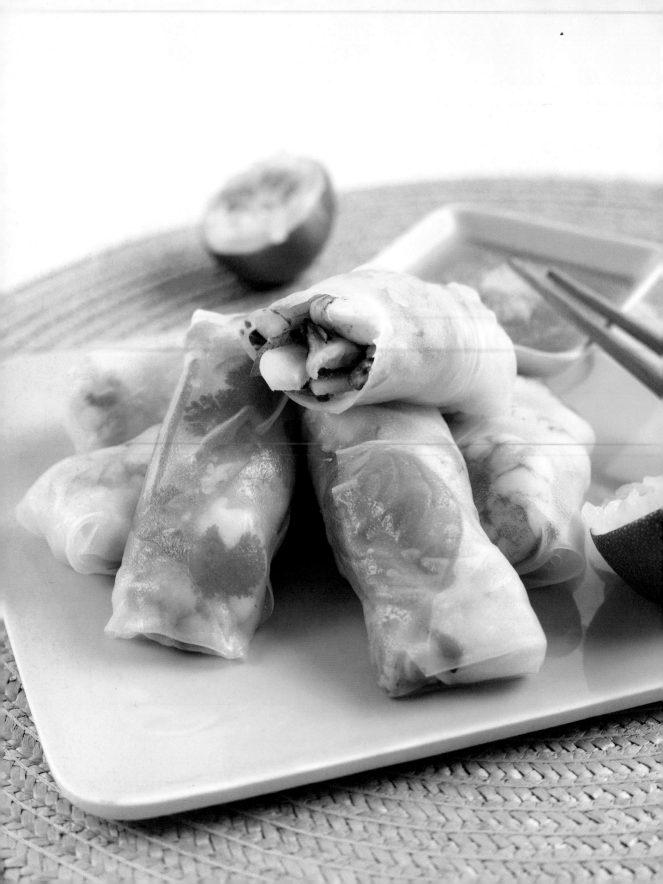

Prawn Rice Paper Spring Rolls

Ingredients

16 x 22cm thin round rice papers
300g large prawns, cooked and peeled
1 bunch of mint, leaves separated
1 bunch of coriander, leaves separated
1 bunch of basil, leaves separated
1 cucumber, peeled, deseeded and cut
  into matchsticks
2 yellow peppers, deseeded and cut
  into matchsticks
400g Chinese mushrooms, lightly pan-fried
  in 1 tablespoon of sesame oil, and cooled
100g cashew nuts, roasted and chopped
1 small bag of rocket
2.5cm piece of fresh ginger, peeled
  and grated

For the dipping sauce
juice of 1 lime
2 tablespoons fish sauce
1 tablespoon rice vinegar

Method

1. Prepare all the ingredients as above and have a bowl of warm water and 2 clean, damp tea towels ready.

2. Soak one of the rice papers in the warm water and lay on the tea towel.

3. Place 3 prawns in the middle with a small pile of the herbs, cucumber, peppers, mushrooms, cashews and a few rocket leaves. Don't overfill or it won't seal it shut.

4. Fold the half nearest to you into the centre, then fold in the ends and repeat with the other side to make a neat roll. Run a damp finger along the edges to seal. Reserve and cover with a damp towel while rolling the rest.

5. Make the dipping sauce by mixing the grated ginger, lime juice, fish sauce and rice vinegar together in a bowl.

6. Dip and enjoy!

Prawn Salad

Ingredients

1 large bag of rocket
2 ripe avocados, sliced
½ cucumber, deseeded and sliced
1 chilli, deseeded and thinly sliced
300g prawns, cooked and peeled
1 bunch of coriander
2 tablespoons coconut oil
juice of ½ lime

Method

1. Layer the rocket on a platter. Top with the avocados, cucumber and chilli. Scatter over the prawns and whole coriander leaves.

2. Drizzle with coconut oil and lime juice and serve immediately.

*remember

The more fresh flavours you put in your food, the better it will taste.

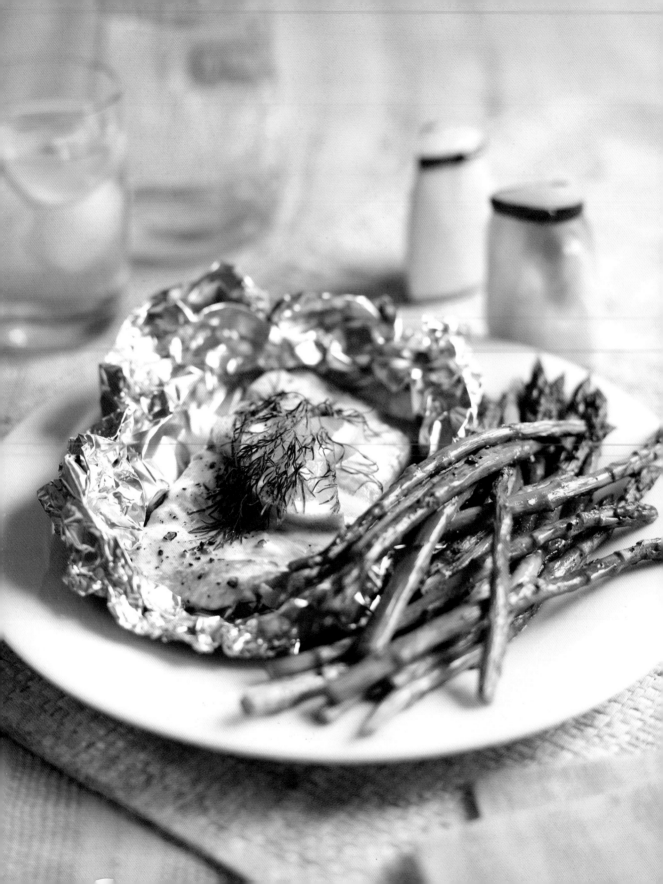

Oven-steamed Salmon with Lemon-roasted Asparagus

Ingredients

4 skinless regular-sized salmon fillets
2 lemons
1 bunch of dill
2 bunches of asparagus
1 tablespoon cold-pressed olive oil
sea salt and pepper

Method

1. Preheat the oven to 200°C/400°F/gas 6.

2. Place the salmon fillets on a large sheet of foil on a baking tray. Season and add a slice of lemon and a sprig of dill to each fillet. Seal the foil parcel and bake in the preheated oven for 12–15 minutes.

3. Meanwhile, place the asparagus in a shallow baking tray, season and drizzle with olive oil and lemon juice. Bake in the oven for 20 minutes.

4. Serve the roasted fish and its juices with the asparagus.

*top tip

Using ingredients such as chilli will add a flavoursome punch to your food.

Squid, Rocket and Chilli Salad

Ingredients

200g mangetout
2 tablespoons sesame oil
juice of 1 lime
800g cleaned squid, cut into 2.5cm strips
2 red chillies, deseeded and thinly sliced
1 large bag of rocket
½ cucumber, deseeded, halved, then cut into 2.5cm slices
1 tablespoon sesame seeds
1 small bunch of coriander, finely chopped

Method

1. Blanch the mangetout in lightly salted boiling water for 3 minutes, drain and run under cold water to cool. Cut lengthways into short ribbons.

2. Make the dressing by whisking together 1 tablespoon of the sesame oil with the lime juice.

3. Heat a non-stick pan, add the remaining sesame oil, then add the squid and chillies. Cook until the squid is no longer translucent, which should take about 5–6 minutes.

4. Arrange the rocket on a serving dish, scatter over the sliced cucumber and mangetout. Add the cooked squid and pour over the dressing. Scatter sesame seeds and chopped coriander over the top.

Ginger-rubbed Prawns with Zingy Mangetout and Broccoli

Ingredients

600g large, raw tiger prawns, peeled
2.5cm piece of fresh ginger, peeled
 and grated
1 red chilli, finely sliced
zest and juice of 2 limes
2 heads of broccoli
400g mangetout
2 tablespoons sesame oil
1 bunch of coriander, chopped

Method

1. Marinate the prawns in the ginger, chilli and half of the lime juice.

2. Blanch the broccoli and mangetout in salted water for about 4 minutes. Drain and toss in the rest of the lime juice, the lime zest and 1 tablespoon of the sesame oil.

3. Heat the remaining sesame oil in a non-stick frying pan and fry the prawns until they turn pink.

4. Serve with the vegetables, a wedge of lime, and the coriander sprinkled over the top.

*top tip
Ginger boosts the immune system and aids digestion.

Yogurt and Harissa Chicken

Ingredients

4 boneless free-range chicken breasts
2 tablespoons rose/plain harissa
2 garlic cloves, crushed
2 tablespoons olive oil
1 bunch of coriander, chopped
100ml organic natural yogurt
rocket leaves, to serve

Method

1. Put the chicken in a bowl, mix with the harissa, garlic, oil and half the coriander. Marinate for about 15 minutes.

2. Preheat the grill to high.

3. Put the chicken breasts on a baking tray and grill for about 6 minutes on each side.

4. Sprinkle over the rest of the coriander and pour on some yogurt and serve with rocket leaves.

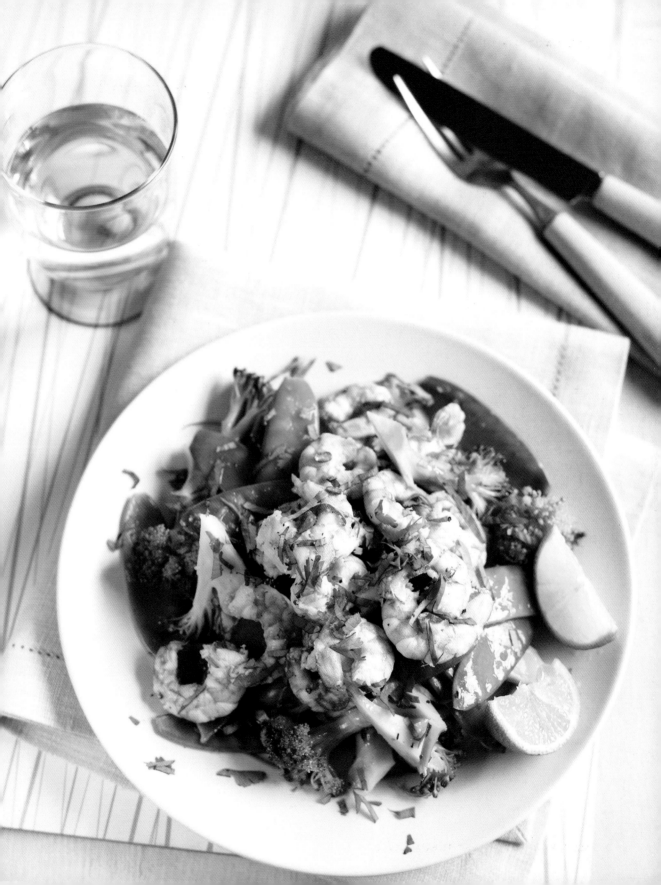

Seared Scallops with Pea Purée and Courgette Ribbons

Ingredients
1kg frozen petit pois
200ml natural organic yogurt
zest and juice of 1 lemon
2 large courgettes
2 tablespoons olive oil
12 fresh scallops, roe removed
salt and pepper

Method
1. Boil the frozen peas, drain, and mix with the salt, pepper, yogurt, lemon juice and zest. Put in a blender and pulse until coarse.

2. Peel the courgettes into ribbons lengthways. Blanch in salted water for 2 minutes, drain, then toss in 1 tablespoon of the olive oil, plus salt and pepper.

3. Heat a non-stick frying pan. Add the remaining olive oil, and sear the scallops for about 30 seconds on each side until opaque.

4. Serve the scallops on the pea purée with a lemon wedge and the courgette ribbons.

Green Bean, Asparagus and Garlic Tortilla

Ingredients
200g green beans, cut into 2.5cm pieces
200g asparagus, cut into 2.5cm pieces
6 free-range eggs
1 tablespoon olive oil
2 garlic cloves, crushed
1 white onion, sliced
salt and pepper

Method:
1. Preheat the grill to high.

2. Blanch the green beans and asparagus in salted water for 2 minutes then drain.

3. Whisk the eggs with salt and pepper

4. Heat the oil in a non-stick frying pan over a medium heat and fry the garlic and onion until soft. Then add the beans and asparagus.

5. Pour the eggs into the pan, making sure they're evenly spread. Use a spatula to pull the edges in, and cook over a medium to low heat for about 10 minutes.

6. Place under the preheated grill, and cook for a further 8 minutes or until golden.

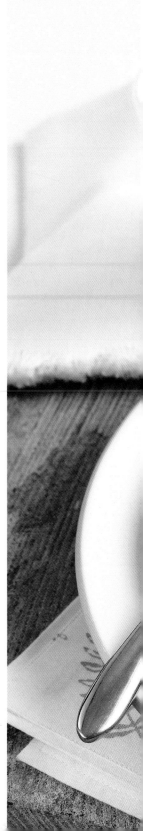

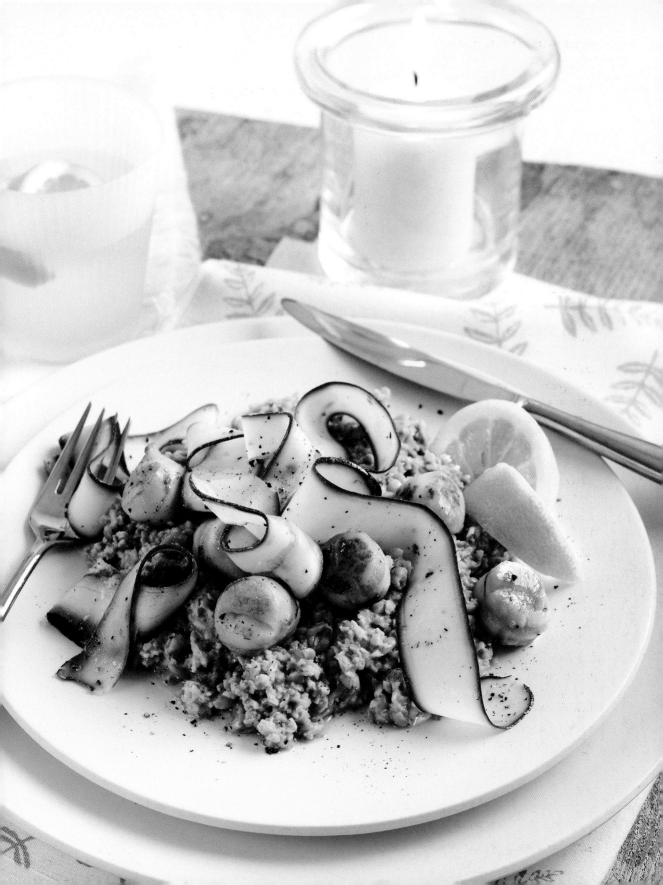

*top tip

Organic vegetables can contain up to twice as many vitamins as non-organic ones.

Yam and Roast Potato Wedges with Lime-yogurt Dip

Ingredients

4 large orange sweet potatoes
4 large wild yams
2 tablespoons olive oil
2 teaspoon cinnamon
2 teaspoon paprika
zest and juice of 1 lime
1 small bunch of coriander, finely chopped
300ml organic natural yogurt
salt and pepper

Method

1. Preheat the oven to 200°C/400°F/gas 6.

2. Cut the sweet potatoes and yams into even wedges. Mix the olive oil, salt and pepper, cinnamon and paprika in a bowl and use this to rub all over the wedgs. Put them on a baking tray and bake for 40–50 minutes or until golden with a crisp skin and soft, fluffy interior.

3. Meanwhile, mix the lime juice and zest with the chopped coriander and yogurt. Serve with the wedges.

Herb-crusted Lamb Cutlets with Tomato, Almond and Green Bean Salad

Ingredients

1 bunch (each) of parsley, mint and basil, finely chopped, plus 1 bunch of basil, left whole
12 lamb cutlets
3 tablespoons olive oil
200g green beans
6 vine tomatoes
juice of 1 lemon
100g flaked almonds, lightly toasted
salt and pepper

Method

1. Preheat the grill to medium.

2. Rub the cutlets with 1 tablespoon of oil and roll in the chopped herbs. Grill the cutlets for about 3–4 minutes on each side.

3. Meanwhile, blanch the green beans in salted water for about 4 minutes.

4. Cut the tomatoes into wedges and toss with the green beans, lemon juice, whole basil leaves, salt and pepper. Sprinkle over flaked almonds and serve with the cutlets.

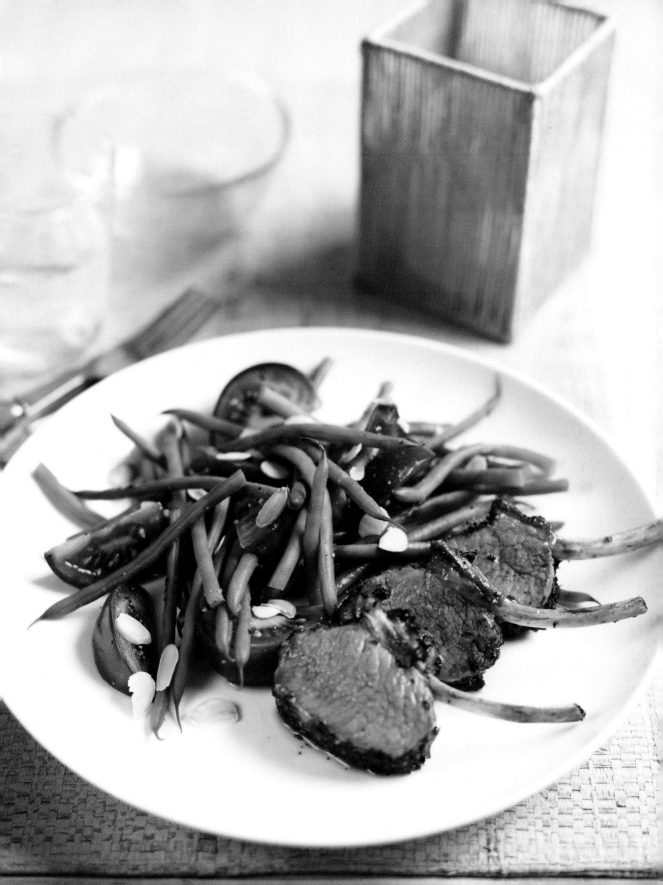

Super Slaw

Ingredients
200ml organic natural yogurt
salt and pepper
2 tablespoons wholegrain mustard
juice of 1 lemon
1 large bunch of kale
1 bag of Brussels sprouts
1 bunch of tarragon, leaves removed
  from stalks
1 bag of baby spinach
100g pumpkin seeds

Method
1. Make the dressing by whisking together the yogurt, a pinch of salt and pepper, mustard and some lemon juice to taste.

2. Very finely slice or shred the kale and Brussels sprouts. Finely chop the tarragon leaves, and place in a large bowl with the spinach, shredded kale, Brussels sprouts and dressing. Sprinkle pumpkin seeds over the top.

Seared Asian Beef Salad with Roast Yam Chips

Ingredients
2 large yams, cut into chips
2 tablespoons olive oil
salt and pepper
2 sirloin steaks
1 tablespoon sesame oil
juice of 1 lime
1 tablespoon rice wine vinegar
1 cucumber, deseeded and cut into
  thin matchsticks
1 red pepper, deseeded and cut into strips
1 yellow pepper, deseeded and cut into strips
1 bag of bean sprouts
1 bag of rocket
1 bag of watercress
1 bag of baby spinach
100g cashew nuts
1 bunch of coriander, leaves removed
  from stalks

Method
1. Preheat the oven to 200°C/400°F/gas 6.

2. Toss the yam chips in 1 tablespoon of the olive oil and some salt and pepper. Place on a baking tray and bake in the preheated oven for about 40 minutes.

3. Heat a griddle pan over a high heat for 4 minutes until hot.

4. Rub the steaks with the remaining olive oil and some salt and pepper. Grill for 4 minutes (or to your liking) on each side. Remove from the grill and leave to rest on a plate.

5. Whisk the sesame oil, lime juice and rice wine vinegar together to make a dressing.

6. Toss all the vegetables together in the dressing and put on a platter. Scatter over cashew nuts.

7. Slice the steaks on an angle, lay over the salad and garnish with coriander leaves.

*top tip
The more nutrients your body consumes, the less hungry you'll feel.

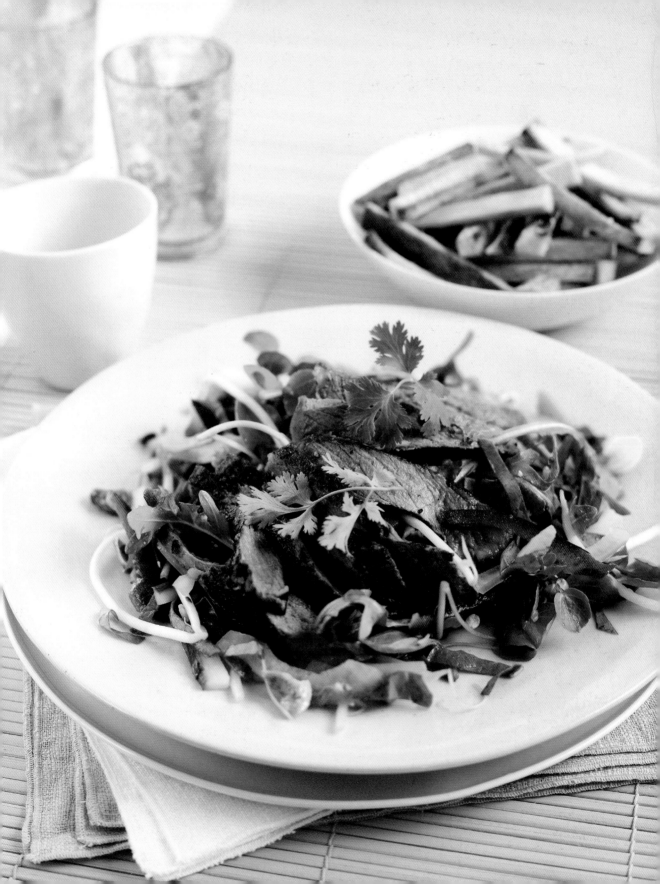

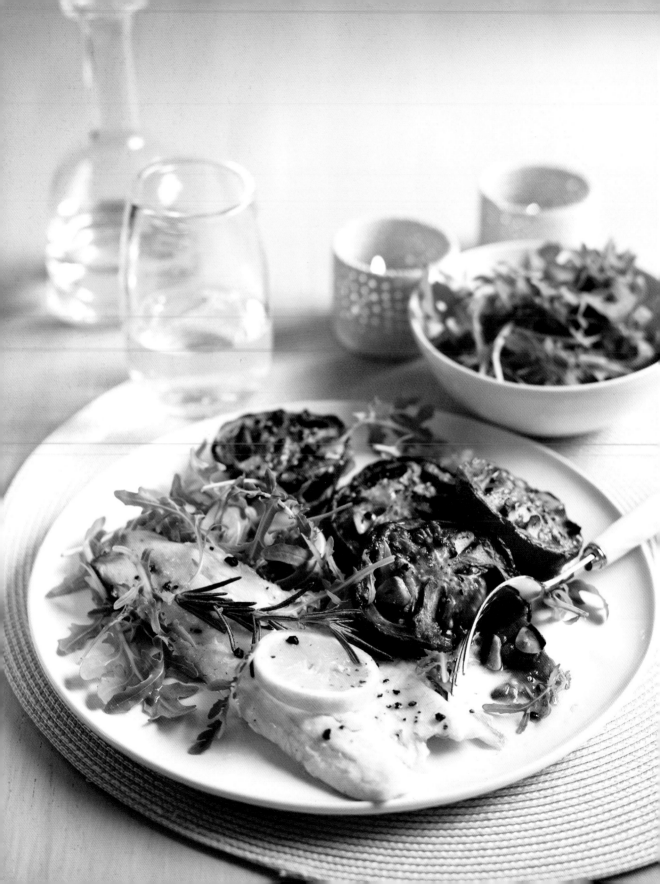

Baked Sea Bass with Roast Tomatoes

Ingredients

8 large vine tomatoes, halved
2 garlic cloves, thinly sliced
2 tablespoons olive oil
salt and pepper
4 sea bass fillets (about 100g each)
1 lemon, cut into 4 slices
4 stems rosemary
200g organic rocket
extra virgin olive oil, to serve

Method

1. Preheat the oven to 200°C/400°F/gas 6.

2. Place the tomato halves on a baking tray. Press garlic slices into them, drizzle over 1 tablespoon of oil and season with salt and pepper. Roast in the preheated oven for 35 minutes.

3. Lay the sea bass fillets on a large sheet of foil on a baking tray. Place 1 slice of lemon and 1 sprig of rosemary on each fillet, drizzle with the remaining oil, season with salt and pepper, seal the foil into a parcel and put in the oven for the last 8 minutes of the tomatoes' cooking time.

4. Serve the fish and tomatoes on a bed of rocket with a drizzle of extra-virgin olive oil.

Warm Anchovy, Broccoli and Chilli Salad

Ingredients

1 head of broccoli
350g tenderstem or purple sprouting broccoli
4 anchovy fillets (from a tin) in olive oil
2 garlic cloves, crushed
1 red chilli, sliced
½ tablespoon dried chilli flakes
2 tablespoons extra-virgin olive oil

Method

1. Blanch both the broccoli in lightly salted water until tender but with a bite (usually about 4–7 minutes).

2. Heat a deep frying pan over a medium heat, add the anchovies together with their oil and mix with the crushed garlic. Mash with a fork to create a paste. Add the sliced chilli and chilli flakes. Add the broccoli to the pan and toss for 2–3 minutes, making sure the broccoli is coated in the anchovy paste.

2. Arrange on a serving plate and drizzle with extra-virgin olive oil.

*it's easy

This salad is an explosion of flavour on your plate, plus it's packed full of nutrients.

Kale has powerful antioxidant properties, plus it's an anti-inflammatory too.

Turkey with Mustard, Sage and Yogurt

Ingredients
2 large, skinless turkey breasts
1 tablespoon olive oil
3 tablespoons grainy mustard
1 bunch of sage, thinly sliced
200ml natural organic yogurt
400g baby spinach
salt and pepper

Method
1. Slice the turkey into thin strips.

2. Heat the oil in a deep frying pan, and cook the turkey until light brown. Add the mustard, sage and yogurt, season, then turn down the heat and simmer for 15–20 minutes.

3. Steam the spinach and serve with the cooked turkey.

Seared Ginger Duck with Wilted Kale and Sesame Seeds

Ingredients
4 small duck breasts, with skin
5cm piece of fresh ginger, peeled and grated
2 garlic cloves, crushed
2 tablespoons sesame oil
2 large bunches of green kale
3 tablespoons sesame seeds
juice of 1 lemon

Method
1. Preheat the oven to 200°C/400°F/gas 6.

2. Score the skin of the duck breasts on an angle and marinate in a bowl with the ginger, garlic and 1 tablespoon of the sesame oil.

3. Heat a griddle or heavy frying pan. Once hot, place the duck breasts (skin side down) in the pan and sear for about 8–10 minutes, or until crisp and browned. Sear on the other side for 4 minutes. Transfer to an ovenproof dish and finish in the preheated oven for about 10 minutes, or until cooked to your liking.

4. In a wok, heat the remaining sesame oil, add the kale and cover with a lid and wilt for about 6–8 minutes. Add the sesame seeds and lemon juice.

5. Slice the duck breasts on an angle and serve on top of the kale.

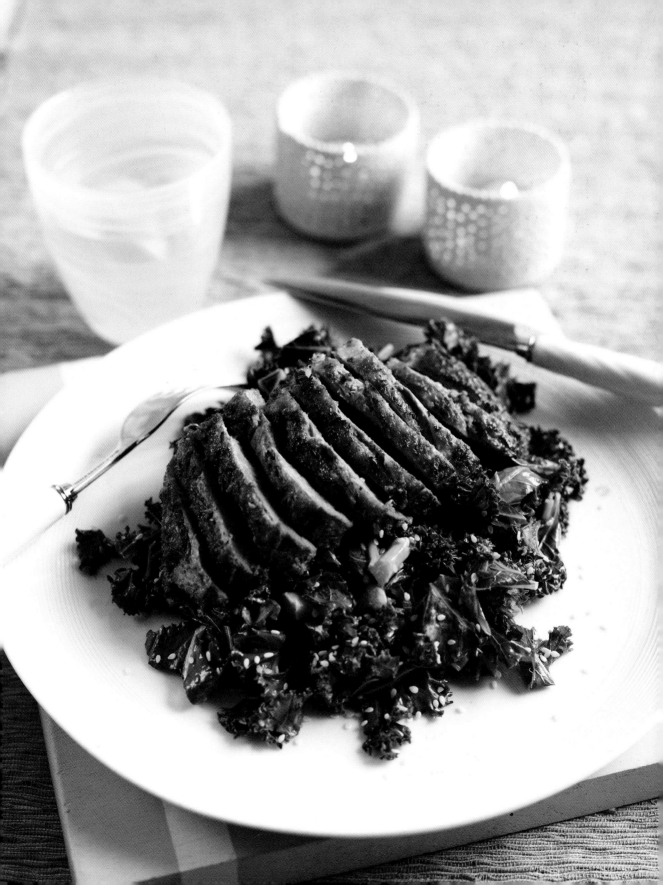

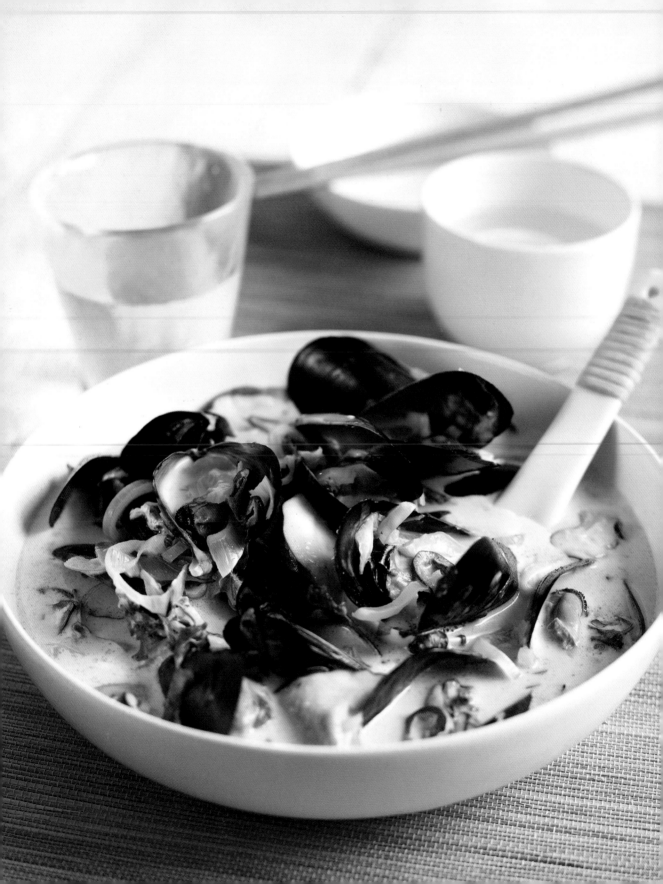

Chilli and Coriander Mussel Broth with Chinese Mushrooms and Bok Choy

Ingredients

1 tablespoon oil
2 white onions, sliced
2 garlic cloves, finely sliced
2 red chillies, deseeded and finely sliced
400ml (1 can) coconut milk
300ml organic fish stock
200g Chinese mushrooms, sliced
32 cleaned, closed mussels
2 heads of bok choy, leaves separated
1 bunch of coriander, leaves picked
  off stalks

Method

1. Heat the oil in a deep saucepan over a medium heat, then fry the onions, garlic and chillies until soft (about 10 minutes).

2. Add the coconut milk and the fish stock, then the mushrooms and mussels. Cover and cook for about 8 minutes or until all the mussels have opened.

3. Add the bok choy and half the coriander and replace the lid for 2 minutes.

4. Throw out any mussels that still haven't opened and serve with the remaining coriander sprinkled over the top.

Moroccan Lamb Tenderloin with Sweet Potato and Cinnamon Mash

Ingredients

1 teaspoon ground cumin
1 teaspoon ground coriander
1 teaspoon ground cinnamon
1 teaspoon ras el hanout (a Moroccan
  dry spice mix)
salt and pepper
2 boneless lamb loin fillets (weighing about
  150g each)
1 tablespoon sherry vinegar
1 tablespoon olive oil
4 orange sweet potatoes
2 tablespoons natural organic yogurt
1 teaspoon cinnamon
1 bunch of fresh coriander, chopped

Method

1. Preheat the oven to 220°C/425°F/gas mark 7.

2. Mix the first 4 spices with salt and pepper.

3. Rub the lamb loins with the sherry vinegar, oil and mixed spices. Place in a baking dish and roast for 30–40 minutes, basting regularly.

4. Peel and cut the sweet potatoes into chunks. Place in a pan of boiling water and cook until soft. Mash the sweet potatoes, then stir in the yogurt and ground cinnamon.

5. Slice the lamb into thick slices and serve on the mash with some of the cooking juices drizzled over the top and a sprinkle of dropped coriander.

CHAPTER 8

THE 6-DAY TUMMY TRANSFORMER

THIS CHAPTER IS ALL ABOUT:

ACHIEVING A FLAT TUMMY IN JUST 6 DAYS
- THAT'S IT!

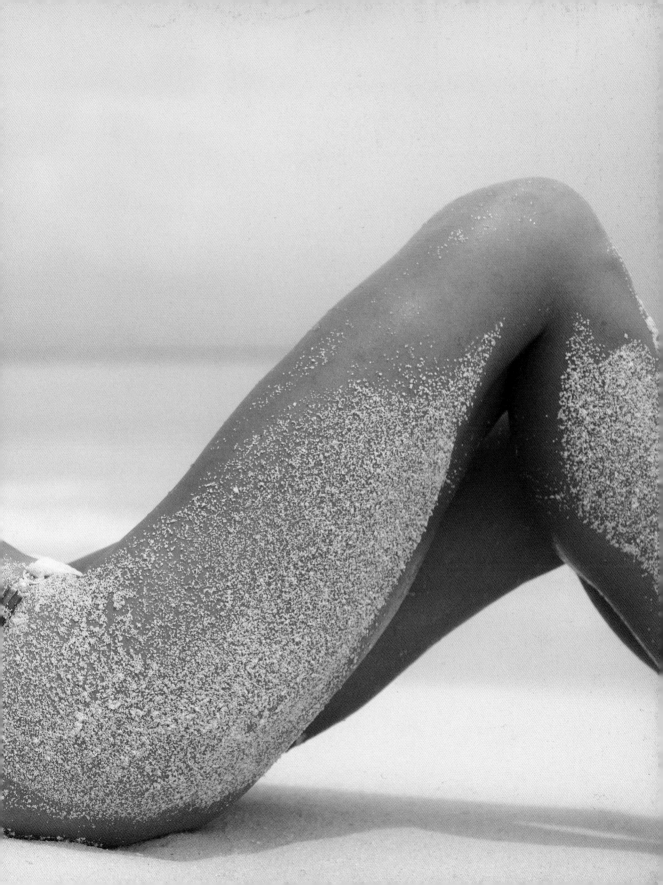

This is tough, but effective. When a client comes to me and says they need to look bikini-ready by the weekend this is what I prescribe. Models use it for photo shoots, and it's also good for holidays, weddings and any other occasion where you want to look your best in as speedy a time as possible.

It isn't dangerous. There's no crash dieting or weird liquid diets involved. It's safe and healthy. But it is tough. You have to stick to the rules religiously if you want to see results. But it only lasts 6 days so it's doable, and best of all, the results are phenomenal. So here it is:

RULES OF THE 6-DAY TUMMY TRANSFORMER

✳ Limit your salt intake – it holds on to water, which causes tummy bloating.

✳ No spicy herbs – chilli can inflame the gut wall and make it stick out.

✳ Water only – unlike the 14-day plan where you can have coffee every day, here you can't. The only caffeine you can have is in green tea, which is so full of antioxidants it helps reduce stress on the body (remember: stress = a fat tummy).

✳ No fat – except a Bodyism fish oil capsule at each meal.

✳ Lean white meat only – that means chicken, turkey and white fish.

✳ All food has to be steamed, baked or grilled with no added oil. Boring, but brilliantly effective in 6 days.

✳ You need to drink at least 2–3 litres of still filtered water a day. Along with all the fibre you're having, this will sweep through your system, cleaning out your bowels and giving a flatter, leaner stomach.

✳ Talking of fibre, you'll need lots of it – it rids the body of toxins and foreign oestrogen (from medication, the environment, etc.).

During the 6-Day Tummy Transformer, you'll be eating around 1500 calories a day. This isn't advisable for pregnant or breastfeeding women. However, most of us can cope perfectly well on this a day as long as it's for short periods of time and we're getting the right amount of vitamins, minerals and nutrients in those 1500 calories. Lean white protein and green vegetables keep you full and provide you with these nutrients, yet they're incredibly low in calories. This isn't the same as surviving on 1000 calories worth of diet cola and low-fat cereal a day. This is the healthy way to do it.

The green vegetables in this 6-day plan have been specifically chosen to help your body become less acidic (remember, less acid = a flatter tummy). This helps your body burn fat faster (especially around the middle). Plus it means fewer toxins in your system, which benefits your waist, tummy, overall health and overall appearance (better skin, hair, etc.). As you won't be eating any complex carbs (such as bread, pasta, rice) your body will constantly be burning fat.

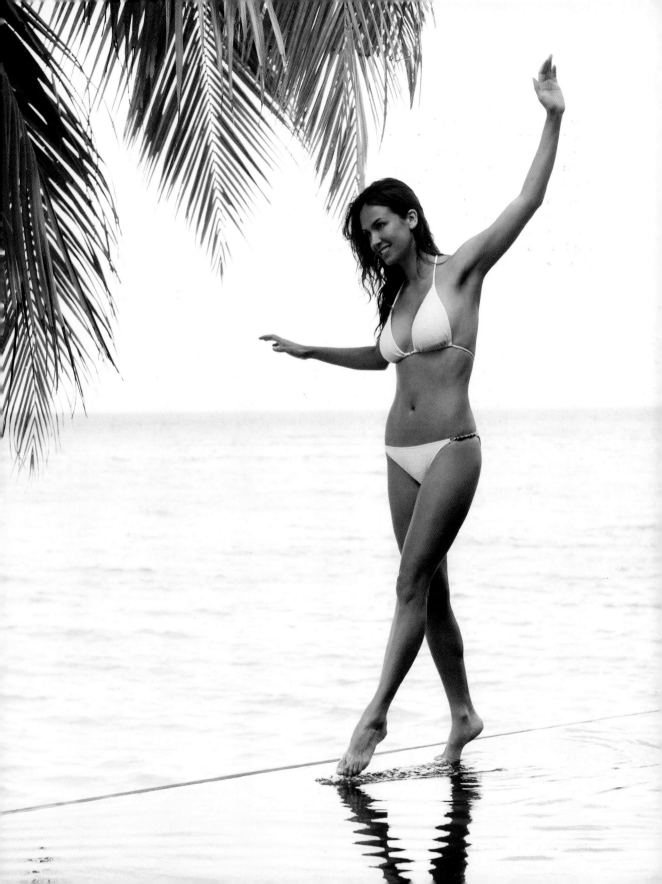

IT'S TOUGH, BORING AND REPETITIVE.

DAY 1

As soon as you wake up: A mug of slightly cooled boiled water with freshly squeezed lemon or lime and 1 scoop of Bodyism Fibre (available at www.bodyism.com).

Breakfast: A 2-egg-white omelette with steamed spinach.

Snack, mid-morning: 100g lean white meat and a quarter of a cucumber.

Lunch: 1 chicken breast with steamed asparagus.

Snack, mid-afternoon: 100g lean white meat and ¼ cucumber, sliced.

Dinner: Steamed cod fillet and steamed green vegetables.

Before bed: 1 scoop of Bodyism Fibre in a glass of water with Body Serenity (available at www.bodyism.com).

Supplements: 3 Bodyism Fish Oils (take 1 after each main meal); 3 Bodyism Multi-vitamins (take one after each meal).

Drinks: 2-3 litres of still, filtered water (try not to drink it too close to mealtimes).

DAY 2

As soon as you wake up: A mug of slightly cooled boiled water with freshly squeezed lemon or lime and 1 scoop of Bodyism Fibre.

Breakfast: 150g turkey breast with steamed spinach.

Snack, mid-morning: 100g lean white meat and a quarter of a cucumber, sliced.

Lunch: 1 chicken breast with steamed green beans.

Snack mid afternoon: 100g lean white meat and ¼ cucumber, sliced.

Dinner: Steamed haddock with steamed green vegetables.

Before bed: 1 scoop of Bodyism Fibre in a glass of water with Body Serenity.

Supplements: 3 Bodyism Fish Oils (take 1 after each main meal); 3 Bodyism Multi-vitamins (take 1 after each meal).

Drinks: 2-3 litres of still, filtered water (try not to drink it too close to mealtimes).

DAY 3

As soon as you wake up: A mug of slightly cooled boiled water with freshly squeezed lemon or lime and 1 scoop of Bodyism Fibre.

Breakfast: 150g turkey breast with steamed kale.

Snack, mid-morning: 100g lean white meat and a quarter of a cucumber, sliced.

Lunch: Baked sea bass with steamed broccoli.

Snack, mid-afternoon: 100g lean white meat and ¼ cucumber, sliced.

Dinner: 1 chicken breast and steamed Brussels sprouts.

Before bed: 1 scoop of Bodyism Fibre in a glass of water with Body Serenity.

Supplements: 3 Bodyism Fish Oils (take 1 after each main meal); 3 Bodyism Multi-vitamins (take 1 after each meal).

Drinks: 2-3 litres of still, filtered water (try not to drink it too close to mealtimes).

BUT IT GETS RESULTS! SO, HERE GOES:

DAY 4

As soon as you wake up: A mug of slightly cooled boiled water with freshly squeezed lemon or lime and 1 scoop of Bodyism Fibre.

Breakfast: A 2-egg-white omelette with purple-sprouting broccoli.

Snack, mid-morning: 100g lean white meat and ¼ cucumber, sliced.

Lunch: 1 chicken breast with steamed asparagus.

Snack, mid-afternoon: 100g lean white meat and ¼ cucumber, sliced.

Dinner: Steamed cod and steamed bok choy.

Before bed: 1 scoop of Bodyism Fibre in a glass of water with Body Serenity.

Supplements: 3 Bodyism Fish Oils (take 1 after each main meal); 3 Bodyism Multi-vitamins (take 1 after each meal).

Drinks: 2–3 litres of still, filtered water (try not to drink it too close to mealtimes).

DAY 5

As soon as you wake up: A mug of slightly cooled boiled water with freshly squeezed lemon or lime and 1 scoop of Bodyism Fibre.

Breakfast: 1 baked chicken breast and steamed green beans.

Snack mid morning: 100g lean white meat and ¼ cucumber, sliced.

Lunch: 1 baked halibut with steamed broccoli.

Snack, mid-afternoon: 100g lean white meat and ¼ cucumber, sliced.

Dinner: 1 grilled chicken breast and steamed asparagus.

Before bed: Body Serenity.

Supplements: 3 Bodyism Fish Oils (take 1 after each main meal); 3 Bodyism Multi-vitamins (take 1 after each meal).

Drinks: 2–3 litres of still, filtered water (try not to drink it too close to mealtimes).

DAY 6

As soon as you wake up: A mug of slightly cooled boiled water with freshly squeezed lemon or lime and 1 scoop of Bodyism Fibre.

Breakfast: 150g turkey breast and steamed spinach.

Snack, mid- morning: 100g lean white meat and ¼ cucumber, sliced.

Lunch: 1 chicken breast with spinach.

Snack, mid-afternoon: 100g lean white meat and ¼ cucumber, sliced.

Dinner: Steamed lemon sole and steamed mangetout.

Before bed: Body Serenity.

Supplements: 3 Bodyism Fish Oils (take 1 after each main meal); 3 Bodyism Multi-vitamins (take 1 after each meal).

Drinks: 2–3 litres of still, filtered water (try not to drink it too close to mealtimes).

YOUR 6-DAY EXERCISE PROGRAMME

STAGE 1

Morning cardio

Why? Short bursts of cardio first thing in the morning will boost fat burning.

When? Monday, Wednesday and Friday mornings.

DETAILS:

1. 3 minutes of brisk walking
2. 2 minutes of jogging (where you can still hold a conversation)
3. 1-minute sprint (as fast as you can)
4. Repeat the above 6 times (the whole thing should take you 24 minutes)
5. Have a 5-minute cool-down (walking and getting your breath back)

*top tip
Lactic acid is a waste product that builds up in your body and makes your muscles feel stiff and sore. When you clear it out you will move more freely and exercise better.

STAGE 2

Fat-burning circuits

Why? This will increase your lean muscle mass, which means you burn fat for longer. Circuits don't raise your cortisol levels in the same way as long stretches of cardio (remember, more cortisol = more fat on your tummy). These exercises are all designed to target your abdominals, especially the lower ones (the ones below your belly button). They also target them from different angles.

When? Monday, Wednesday and Friday evenings.

DETAILS:

Monday evening
Do each exercise one after the other, then start again, a total of 3 times. Have a 45-second rest after each completed circuit:

1. 10 push-ups (see p. 70)
2. 10 squats with a 30-second hold after the last rep (where your thighs are parallel to the ground) (see p.72)
3. 10 squat jumps
4. 10 triceps dips
5. 10 lunges
6. 10 (each leg, so 20 in total) split-squat jumps
7. 10 abdominal leg lowerings
8. 1 minute of jumping Jacks

Wednesday evening
Do each exercise one after the other, then start again, a total of 3 times. Have a 45-second rest after each

completed circuit:

1. 12 squats with a 30-second hold after the last rep (where thighs are parallel to the ground)
2. 12 push-ups
3. 12 squat jumps
4. 12 reverse lunges
5. 12 triceps dips
6. 12 (each leg, so 24 in total) split-squat jumps
7. 12 side-bridge holds with leg raise
8. 2 minutes of jumping Jacks

Friday evening
Do each exercise one after the other, then start again, a total of 5 times. Have a 60-second rest after each completed circuit:

1. 15 squats with a 30-second hold after last the rep (where thighs are parallel to the ground)
2. 15 push-ups
3. 15 squat jumps
4. 15 forward lunges
5. 15 triceps dips
6. 15 (each leg, so 30 in total) split-squat jumps
7. 15 front bridges
8. 2 minutes of jumping Jacks

Resistance training

Note: you'll need two dumbbells for these exercises – anything between 1 and 5kg is OK, depending on your strength and fitness levels.

Why? The increase in weight during exercise means more muscles need to work, which means more lean muscle, which means a flatter stomach. Plus, when your arms are raised above your head holding weights it requires so much stability that your abs get a huge boost.

When? Tuesday and Thursday evenings.

DETAILS:

Tuesday evening

Do each exercise one after the other, then start again, a total of 5 times. Have a 60-second rest after each completed circuit.

You will need: dumbbell or additional weights.

1. 12 dumbbell overhead squats
2. 12 push-ups with rotation
3. 12 squat jumps
4. 12 split squats to press
5. 12 dumbbell bent-over rows
6. 12 reverse lunges to curl
7. 12 burpies
8. 2 minutes of jumping Jacks

Thursday evening

Do each exercise one after the other, then start again, a total of 15 times. Have a 60-second rest after each completed circuit.

You will need: two dumbbells or additional weights.

1. 15 dumbbell overhead squats
2. 15 push-ups with rotation
3. 15 squat jumps
4. 15 split squats to press
5. 15 dumbbell bent-over rows
6. 15 reverse lunges to curl
7. 15 burpies
8. 2 minutes of jumping Jacks

Day 6
AFTER 5 DAYS OF EXERCISING EVERY DAY, YOU NEED TO REST. THIS WILL LET YOUR BODY REGENERATE.

THE EXERCISES
– HOW TO DO THEM!

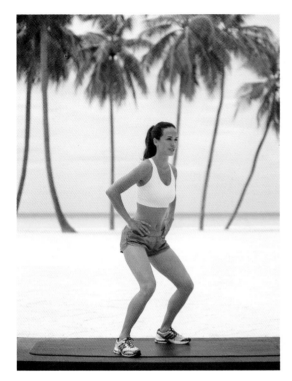

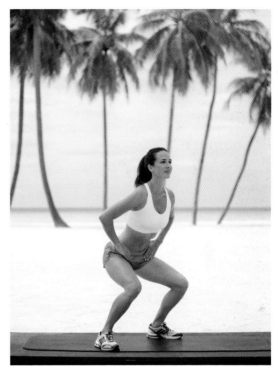

Squat jumps

✳ Start off in a squat position (above) and slowly lower yourself, so your thighs are at least parallel to the ground.

✳ Jump up, and as you come up, land with soft feet and your back in the squat position.

✳ Make sure your knees don't knock in.

*remember
This will burn, however
if you feel pain in your
back or joints, stop.

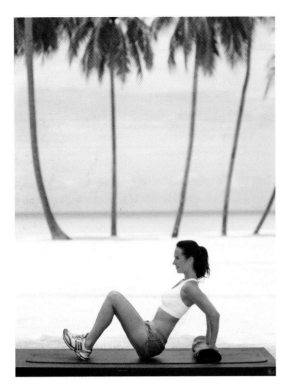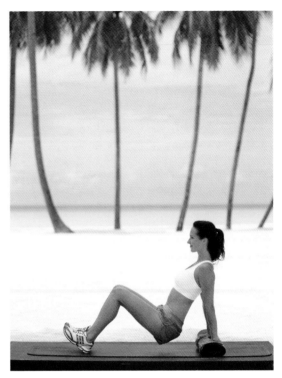

Triceps dips

✳ Start off holding a bench or whatever you can find with your feet slightly elevated (as shown). Set the core and then slowly lower yourself by bending from the elbows so they go backwards and remain close to your sides.

✳ Once your forearms have touched your biceps, straighten your arms back to the start position.

✳ Ensure that you keep your chest up and you look straight ahead and not down.

*reminder
No more excuses! These exercises
can be done anywhere, anytime.

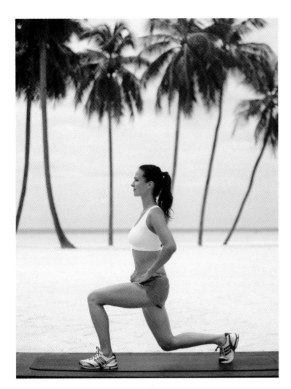
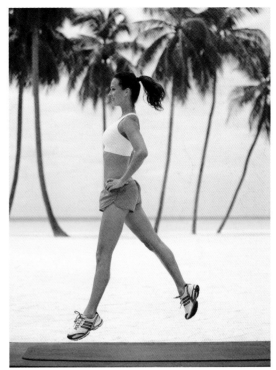

Lunges

✳ Stand with perfect posture with your hands on your hips.

✳ Both feet should face forwards with straight front shins and be hip-width apart.

✳ Contract your stomach muscles.

✳ Lower your body by bending your back knee (your back knee should just touch the floor).

✳ Push up, putting your weight through the heel of your front foot back to the start position.

Lunge jumps

✳ Start off in the split-squat position (see above), then slowly lower yourself down and as you rise up, jump.

✳ Slowly and softly land back in the split-squat position.

✳ Make sure your legs don't creep in, and they stay the same distance apart at all times.

Jumping jacks

✳ Stand with your feet together and your arms raised above your head and set your core.

✳ Bend your knees and jump, moving your feet apart until they are wider than your shoulders. Simultaneously lower your arms.

✳ Keep your knees bent while you jump again, bringing your feet together and your arms back to your sides.

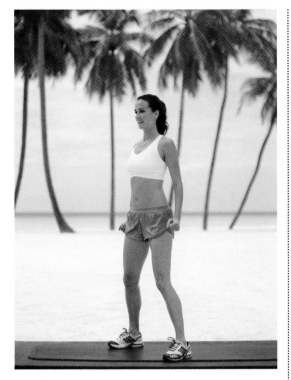

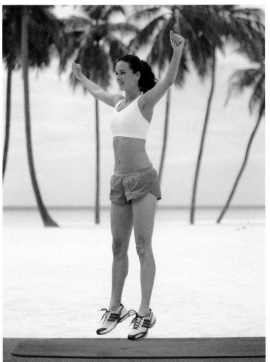

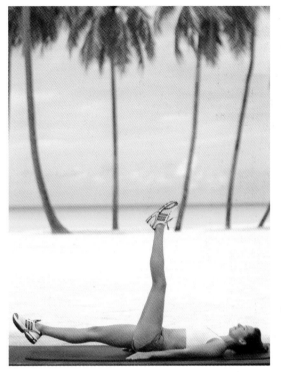

Abdominal leg lowering

✳ Lie on your back with your legs straight up in front of you at right angles to the floor.

✳ Slowly tighten your abs and rotate your pelvis slightly back and down.

✳ Slowly lower one leg, so the thigh is perpendicular to the floor and then switch legs.

*top tip
If your lower back hurts, place a small rolled towel underneath (if it still hurts, stop).

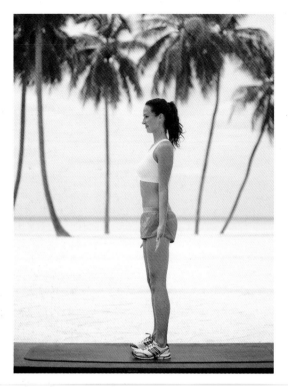

Reverse lunges

✳ Stand with perfect posture, palms and both feet facing out.

✳ Feet should be hip-width apart.

✳ Set the core.

✳ Step back with one leg. Your front shin should be straight and perpendicular to the floor.

✳ Push up with your back leg returning to the standing position.

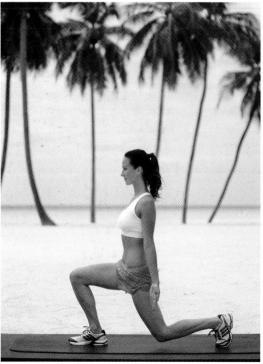

Side-bridge holds
with leg raise (opposite page)

✳ Lie on your side with your elbow under your shoulder and your legs straight and on top of each other.

✳ Bridge up so the weight of your body is on your forearm and feet.

✳ Slowly lift your leg up about 30cm towards the sky, then slowly return to the bridge position.

✳ Your body should remain still in the bridge position at all times.

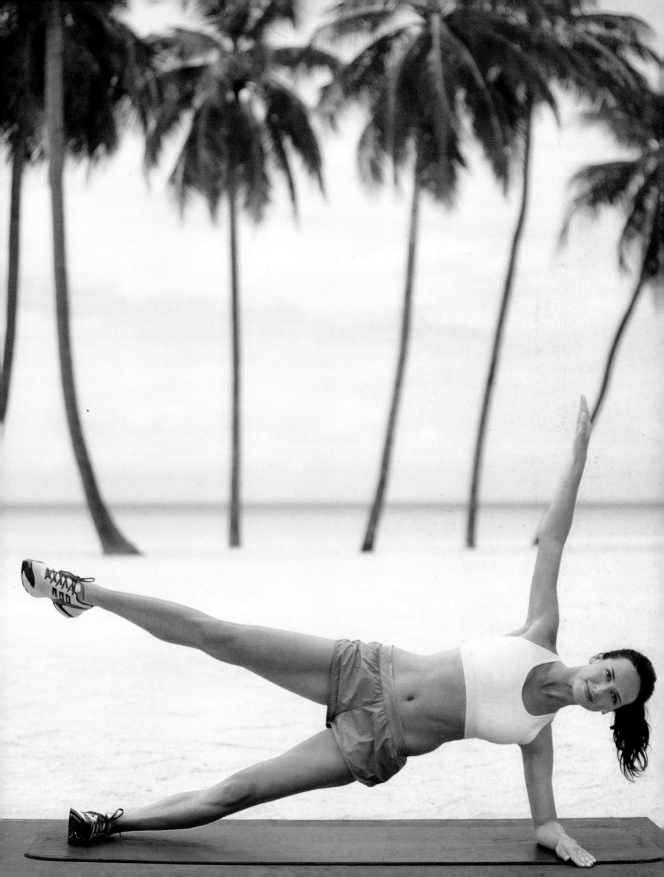

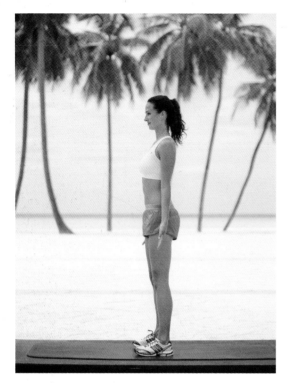

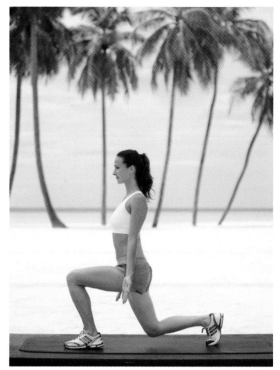

Forward lunges

✳ Stand with perfect posture with palms and both feet facing out.

✳ Feet should be hip-width apart.

✳ Set the core.

✳ Step forward with one leg (as shown). Your front shin should be straight and perpendicular to the floor.

✳ Push up and back with your front leg returning to standing position.

Front bridge
– also known as a plank

✳ Lie face down on the floor with your forearms and elbows touching the floor, and with your hips and legs on the ground.

✳ Raise your body, hips and legs and toes off the floor and set the core, keeping your head aligned with your upper back and hips.

✳ Imagine a straight line from your head to your ankles.

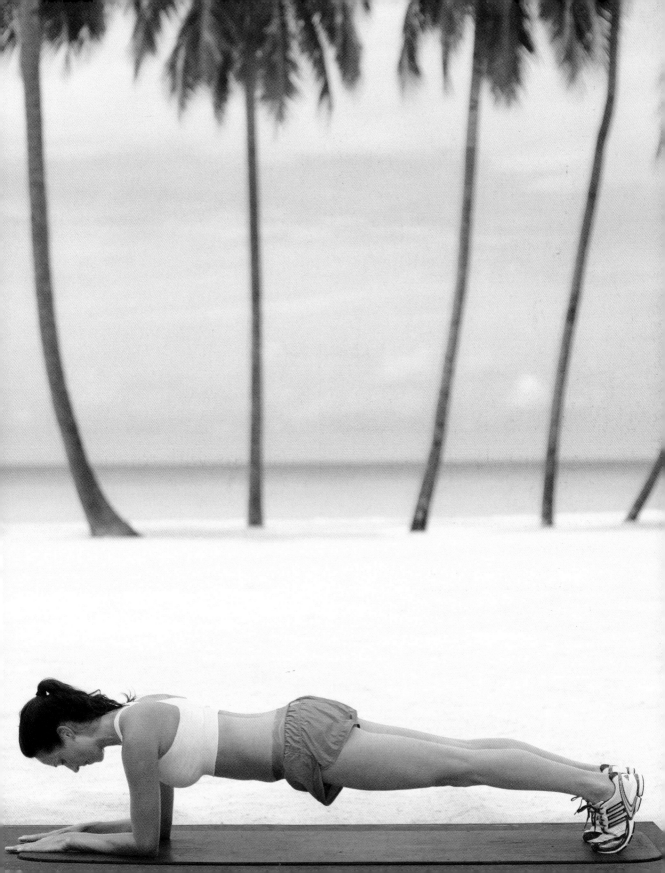

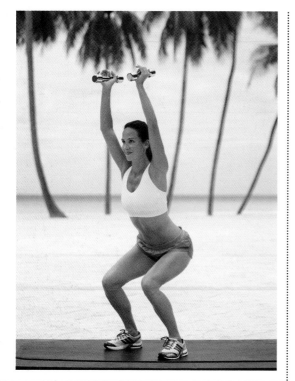

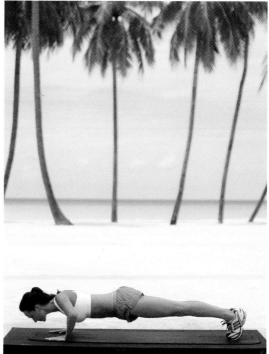

Dumbbell overhead squats

✳ Squat while holding your weights above your head in line with your ears.

✳ Slowly squat down, so your thighs are parallel to the floor, keeping your arms above your head.

✳ As you come back up from the squat make sure that the weights don't come down in front of your head.

Push-ups with rotation

✳ Get into the push-up position. Set your hands one and a half shoulder-widths apart and in line with your nipples, not your shoulders. Keep your legs straight and your weight distributed through your hands and toes.

✳ Keep your ears, shoulders and hips in alignment.

✳ Contract your stomach muscles.

✳ Lower yourself so your nose almost touches the ground, keeping your body straight, then lift yourself back up to the start position.

✳ Once you reach the top position, rotate on your side so that all your body weight is on one arm and both feet.

✳ Hold for 1 second and then return to the start position.

✳ Remember to keep your head up and belly button drawn in.

✳ Breathe out as you push up to the start position, and breathe in as you lower yourself down.

*top tip

Remember why you are doing this
– the results will be amazing!

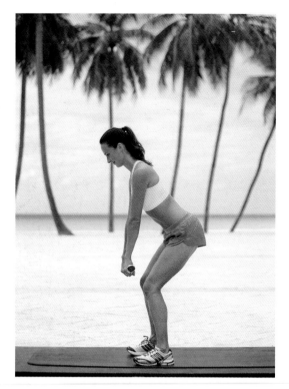 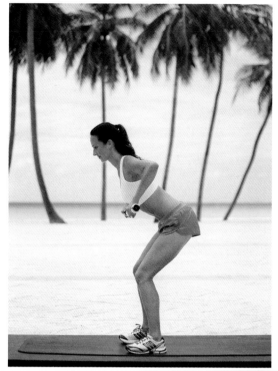

Dumbbell bent-over rows

✳ Start off holding dumbbells in each hand, fists facing forwards; set your stance in an athletic position (with knees slightly bent and back in postural alignment as shown).

✳ Slowly contract your abdominals and shoulder blades and row the dumbbells to your chest.

✳ Slowly lower, ensuring correct posture is maintained.

Split squats to press (opposite)

✳ Stand with perfect posture and both feet facing out.

✳ Feet should be hip-width apart, with straight front shin.

✳ Set the core.

✳ Hold the weights out as shown at shoulder level.

✳ Lower your body by bending your back knee which should just touch the floor.

✳ Push up, putting weight through the heel of the front foot to a standing position.

✳ As you push up to a standing position, complete the press by pushing the weights above your head.

*top tip
These two exercises are a brilliant way of improving your posture and burning fat.

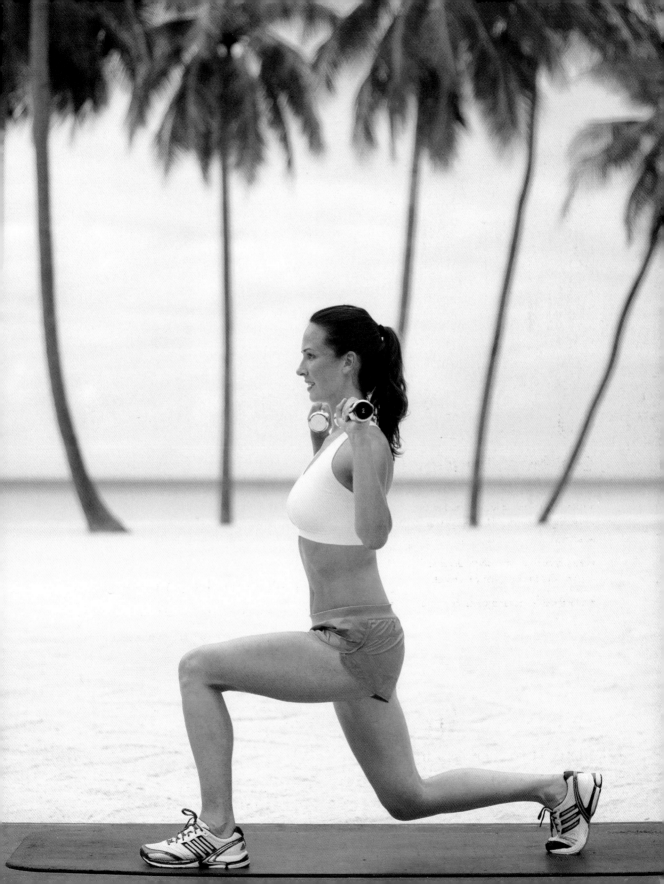

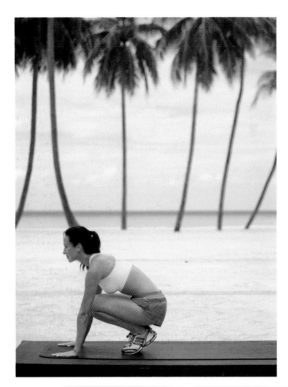
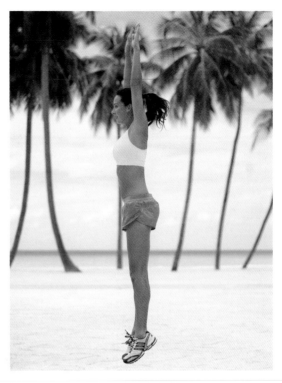

Burpies

✳ Start in a push-up position with your weight equally distributed between your hands and feet.

✳ Jump your feet towards your hands and then stand straight up, your hands in the air and jump. As you land, ensure that your weight is equally distributed on each foot and that your landing is soft.

✳ Once you have finished the jump, place your hands on the floor beside your feet and then jump your feet back into the original push-up position, keeping your back straight when jumping back and your abs tight.

*top tip

Always remember your body loves to move – so get moving and have fun!

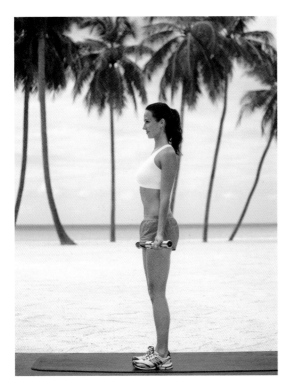

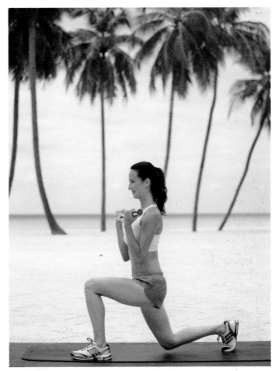

Reverse lunges to curl

✳ Set up with perfect posture, holding dumbbells in each hand.

✳ Both feet should face out and hip-width apart.

✳ Set the core.

✳ Step back with one leg; your front shin should be straight and perpendicular to the floor.

✳ Push up with the back leg, returning to a standing position, then perform a biceps curl by curling your hands towards your shoulders.

CHAPTER 9

FLAT TUMMY FOREVER!

THIS CHAPTER WILL HELP YOU:

1. DISCOVER HOW ELLE MACPHERSON HAS KEPT HER STOMACH FLAT AT EVERY AGE

2. MAKE THE RIGHT FOOD CHOICES TO KEEP A FLAT STOMACH FOR LIFE

Now I've told you everything you need to know about having a flat stomach, I hope you take it all on board and stick to as many of my Clean & Lean rules as you can. Remember, you don't have to stick to every single rule religiously. I understand that at times you're going to want a glass of wine, or a chocolate bar, or to go without exercise for a week or two. And that's absolutely fine. Just stick to my Clean & Lean rules the majority of the time, and you will have a flat stomach forever. One lady who has had a flat stomach forever is my long-time friend Elle Macpherson. I've been training her for over 10 years, and she wrote the foreword for my first book, The Clean & Lean Diet. Here she explains how she has kept her stomach flat, even after 2 children, in her 20s, 30s and 40s.

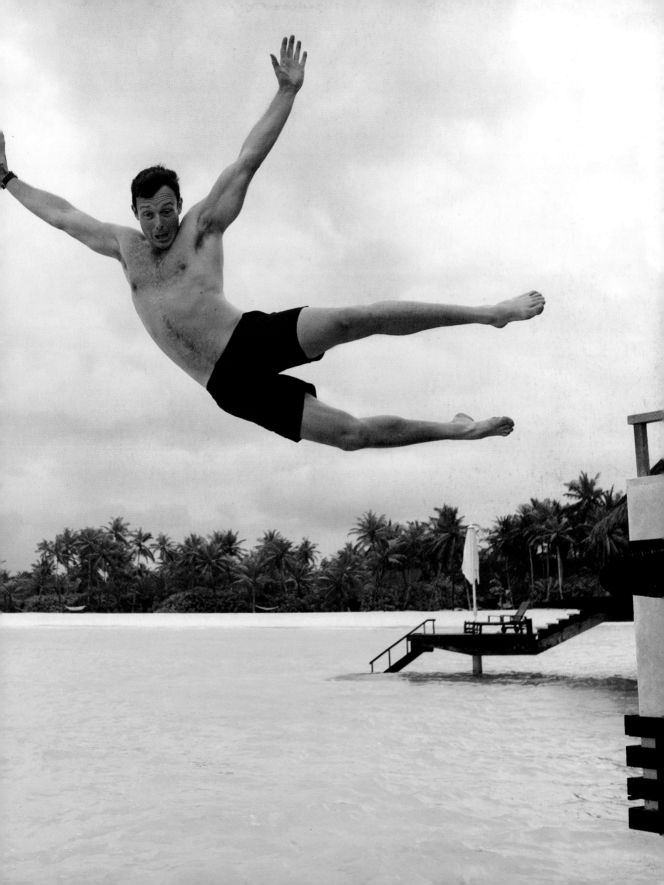

Elle Macpherson

It's been over 15 years since my first meeting with James. We're still friends and I still use his Clean & Lean philosophy to this day. Back then, I hadn't yet had children and found it reasonably easy to keep in athletic shape with a flat stomach. I worked out with James and we were able to keep strong and toned with his mix of Clean & Lean diet ideas, supplements and exercises.

~

Then I had my 2 boys and, like most women who have children, my body changed and the amount of time I had to spend exercising reduced dramatically. As my heart grew with love for my boys, my proportions changed but James rose to the challenge and devised new exercises to tone and flatten the stomach and waist area. Plus he tweaked his diet advice according to my age and lifestyle. He knew I was a busy working mother who had to slot my 'keeping in shape' time around my family and business commitments, and created bespoke diets and fun exercise plans for each stage of my life. I believe my body reflects my lifestyle and even my mindset; it's about having a healthy attitude, appreciating life and being self-loving and responsible. What works for me is a balanced approach, which results in a healthy, vibrant and strong body. I choose not to undermine myself with quick fixes or make life miserable with drastic regimes and hours pounding my body. All I need is the right information and the motivation to do what's required.

~

I've worked closely with James over the years and we have evolved into a really powerful and effective team. I'm healthy and happy and so is he. But here's the thing, as I get older my body and metabolism are also changing. What worked for me in my 20s and 30s doesn't work for me now. But as always, we have been able to work together to find a solution; powerful little nutritional tweaks, along with amazing stress-relieving and body-energising supplements really accelerate the process and we actually have had fun creating this blueprint for a flat tummy.

~

The programme works without punishing my body with gruelling routines. It is a holistic approach based on science and intelligence. The supplements help fine-tune things and make it that little bit easier to get in shape and stay that way, and they taste good so I feed my soul as well. Check out his wife on the cover. She's beautiful, and a true product of a clean & lean life. I hope this book can help you make a profound and powerful transformation in your life.

Elle Macpherson for Australian suncare brand Invisible Zinc. Picture Justin Smith, supplied courtesy of Invisible Zinc.

The programme
works without
punishing my body
with gruelling routines.
It is a holistic approach
based on science
and intelligence.

FINALLY, here are some Bad, Better, Best columns. I give these to all my clients and encourage them

BAD	BETTER	BEST
White sugar	Brown sugar	Manuka honey
Biscuits	Piece of fruit	Piece of fruit and some nuts
Low-fat yogurt	Organic yogurt with fruit and honey	Live organic yogurt with nuts
Candy Bar	Cereal bar	A handful of raw nuts
Soft fizzy drink	Fruit juice	Still, filtered water
Store-bought cake	Fresh cake from a baker	Home-made cake, made with fruit as the sweetener and no white sugar.
Biscuits – full of salt, sugar and bad fat	Oat cakes with nut butter	Rice cakes with turkey and avocado – the perfect blend of proteins, carbs and good fats
Chocolate bar	Fresh fruit and nuts	Raw vegetable with some avocado
Croissant – zero fibre and full of fat	Muffin from a health food store	Raw vegetables with a little organic hummus – loads of fibre, vitamins and minerals
Instant coffee	Espresso	Espresso with organic cream
Black tea	Green tea	Caffeine-free herbal tea – peppermint, camomile etc.
Milk chocolate (chocolate contains caffeine, so avoid it in the evenings)	Dark chocolate – more cocoa satisfies your chocolate craving sooner	Dark chocolate with nuts – the added protein slows the digestion of the sugar preventing an energy crash
Fizzy cola (any brand)	Caffeine-free energy drink – less artificial flavours and sugar	Fruit smoothie
Instant hot drinks – tea, coffee, hot chocolate – processed and full of junk	Espresso with double cream – the cream slows the effects of the caffeine	Caffeine-free herbal tea
Beer – packed with sugar, yeast and alcohol	Organic beer – less pesticides and additives meaning less stress on your liver (meaning a cleaner system)	Vodka, mineral water and a squeeze of lemon or lime – Grey Goose vodka has the least chemicals.
Wine – packed with sugar, yeast and alcohol	Organic wine – see above	Gin and tonic with fresh lime – a clean, yeast-free spirit with minimal calories

to pick foods from the Best column as often as possible... so read, remember and have a flat stomach for life!

BAD	BETTER	BEST
Alco-pop – packed with sugar and alcohol	Vodka and juice (from concentrate) – a lot less sugar	Vodka and freshly squeezed juice
White wine – packed with sugar, yeast and alcohol	White wine spritzer – less sugar and less alcohol	Vodka and mineral water with fresh lemon or lime
Beer – packed with sugar, yeast and alcohol	White wine – less sugar than beer	Red wine – has some antioxidant properties
Cocktails with cola mixers – ie, Long Island Iced Tea – packed with sugar, alcohol and caffeine	Cocktails with fruit mixers – less bad sugars and less calories	Mocktails – non-alcoholic cocktails made with fresh juice
Vodka with energy drink – that caffeine places your internal organs under stress	Vodka and lemonade	Vodka and mineral water with a squeeze of fresh lemon or lime
Shots with a milky liqueur – packed with sugar, dairy and calories	Single shot of clear spirit – less sugar, plus one poison instead of several	Avoid shots altogether!
Malibu and cola – sugar with more sugar, plus caffeine and alcohol	Malibu and pineapple juice – some natural sugars but still a fat bomb	Vodka with a fruit smoothie – clean spirit with nutrients and a little bit of fibre. Sip it slowly and stop at one
Packaged meal with no protein (such as an all-pasta dish) – packed with carbs, sugar, salt and bad fats – and it will leave you hungry because of the lack of protein	Packaged meal with protein (ie, chicken or fish) in it – a step in the right direction	A fresh packaged meal with protein, vegetables and nuts or seeds that can be steamed – not easy to find but when you have no time or energy to make food this is by far the best
Salami – the left over parts of the animal, this is heavily processed and packed with salt	Slice of ham – at least you know what animal it is!	Ham with hummus and avocado – a complete snack of protein, carbs and fats
Salad dressing – packed with sugar, salt and bad fats – if your salad feels too dull, add olive oil, lemon juice or herbs. Clean and Lean flavours!	Balsamic vinegar and olive oil – offers a great flavour and good fats that help fill you up making it a more complete dish	Cold pressed extra virgin olive oil – the least processed of all oils. It's got the most nutrients and the most flavour
Tinned soup	Tub of soup	Organic soup with some protein in it eg. Chicken soup
Ketchup	Pesto	Fresh mashed avocado
White bread	Whole-wheat bread	Rye bread
Wheat-based cereal (check the ingredients)	Oat-based muesli mix with nuts	Half an avocado on a couple of wheat-free oatcakes

INDEX